PREVENTION.

WOMEN'S
HEALTH TODAY
2003

PREVENTION

WOMEN'S HEALTH TODAY 2003

The New Science Behind Weight Loss, Self-Care Remedies, Food Supplements, and Medical Breakthroughs

The Editors of
PREVENTION Magazine

RODALE

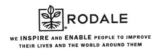

RODALE
WE INSPIRE AND ENABLE PEOPLE TO IMPROVE
THEIR LIVES AND THE WORLD AROUND THEM

FOR PRODUCTS & INFORMATION
WWW.RODALESTORE.COM
WWW.PREVENTION.COM
(800) 848-4735

About *Prevention* Health Books

The editors of *Prevention* Health Books are dedicated to providing you with authoritative, trustworthy, and innovative advice for a healthy, active lifestyle. In all of our books, our goal is to keep you thoroughly informed about the latest breakthroughs in natural healing, medical research, alternative health, herbs, nutrition, fitness, and weight loss. We cut through the confusion of today's conflicting health reports to deliver clear, concise, and definitive health information that you can trust. And we explain in practical terms what each new breakthrough means to you, so you can take immediate, practical steps to improve your health and well-being.

Every recommendation in *Prevention* Health Books is based upon reliable sources, including interviews with qualified health authorities. In addition, we retain top-level health practitioners who serve on the Rodale Books Board of Advisors to ensure that all of the health information is safe, practical, and up-to-date. *Prevention* Health Books are thoroughly fact-checked for accuracy, and we make every effort to verify recommendations, dosages, and cautions.

The advice in this book will help keep you well informed about your personal choices in health care—to help you lead a happier, healthier, and longer life.

Notice

This book is intended as a reference volume only, not as a medical manual. The information given here is designed to help you make informed decisions about your health. It is not intended as a substitute for any treatment that may have been prescribed by your doctor. If you suspect that you have a medical problem, we urge you to seek competent medical help.

Mention of specific companies, organizations, or authorities in this book does not imply endorsement by the publisher, nor does mention of specific companies, organizations, or authorities in the book imply that they endorse the book.

Internet addresses and telephone numbers given in this book were accurate at the time the book went to press.

Board of Advisors

Contents

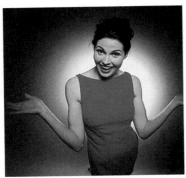

LOOK GREAT!
It's easier than you think.
PAGE 2

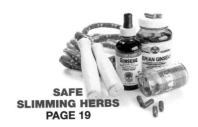

**SAFE
SLIMMING HERBS**
PAGE 19

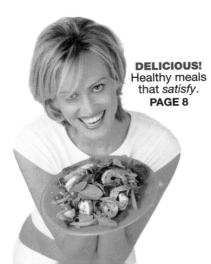

DELICIOUS!
Healthy meals
that *satisfy*.
PAGE 8

PART **TWO**

Quickie Workouts— Fast Results!

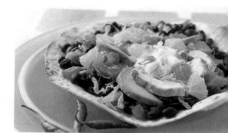

FAST FIX
Veggies as good
as dessert!
PAGE 32

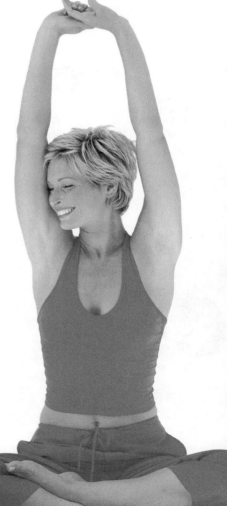

REACH OUT
Energize mind and body!
PAGE 72

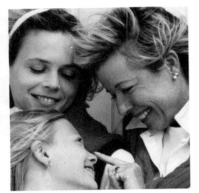

GENETICS
Your key to future health.
PAGE 82

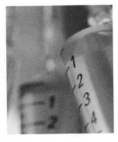

**NEW
ARTHRITIS
FIGHTERS
PAGE 110**

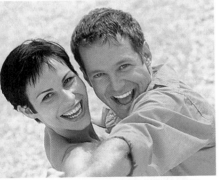

CANCER FREE
Cut your risks—today.
PAGE 96

PART **THREE**

Safeguard Your Health

PART **FOUR**
Mammograms, Menopause, and More

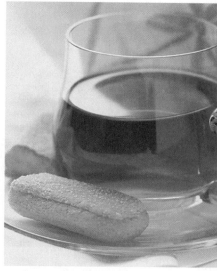

SLEEP BETTER
This brew can help!
PAGE 142

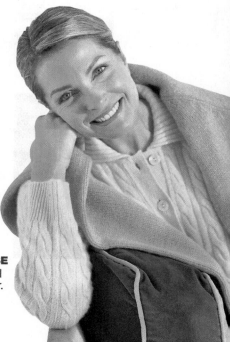

MENOPAUSE
What to tell
your doctor.
PAGE 152

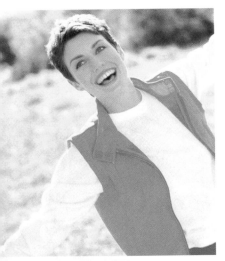

ENERGIZE
9 tips to get you going!
PAGE 156

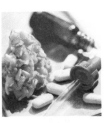

**FIGHT
COLDS
NATURALLY**
PAGE 164

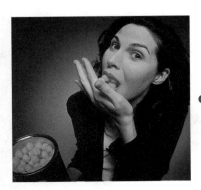

GAINING WEIGHT?
You may have
the Body Blues.
PAGE 177

PART **FIVE**

Everyday Health Boosters

PART **SIX**

Soothe Your Soul

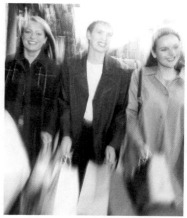

ZAP STRESS
Friendships
are key.
PAGE 193

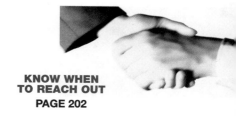

**KNOW WHEN
TO REACH OUT**
PAGE 202

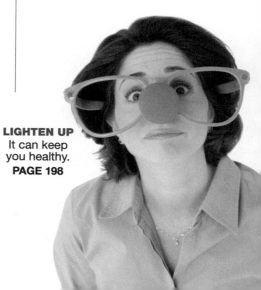

LIGHTEN UP
It can keep
you healthy.
PAGE 198

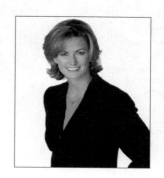

INTRODUCTION
Get Fit, Firm, and Healthy— in Just Minutes a Day!

First, let me just say that I know you're a busy woman. You've got work, family, friends, and the usual household stuff to juggle. It's not easy—I know, because I'm in the same boat!—so before we go any further, give yourself a big pat on the back for all the things you already do! Now, give yourself *another* back-pat for picking up this book, because that means you're motivated to slim down, firm up, eat right, live well, and take good care of yourself. And I'm going to tell you a little secret: *This year, it's easier than ever to do just that!*

This edition of *Women's Health Today* was written with busy women such as you in mind. All of the tips that follow are simple, speedy, and realistic—no major lifestyle changes required. In short, you get to keep living your life—only at the end of the day, you'll look and feel better than you ever dreamed possible!

For instance, our weight loss program will show you how to drop a whole dress size in just 4 weeks, simply by learning a new trick for filling your plate with food. (Yes, I did say *filling*.) Looking to firm up? Our strength-training program provides results in just 8 minutes in the morning, and our walking workout takes less than half of your lunch break!

You'll also find cutting-edge advice on preventing cancer, high cholesterol, diabetes, heart disease, and other serious health conditions, so they won't interfere with your busy life. We've even provided simple tips for making the most of every day by doubling your energy, spending some time on yourself, and getting better sleep when your head finally hits the pillow at night.

Best of all, at the end of each section, you'll find a handy at-a-glance checklist to help you keep your new healthy habits on track with a minimum of effort.

The great news? I know these tips work—and I know how easy they are to implement. With the help of this book, I've lowered my cholesterol, firmed my abs, and learned how to find leisure time in the midst of endless magazine deadlines and motherhood obligations. Now if you'll excuse me, it's time for me to turn off my cell phone and read a good book. Won't you join me?

Catherine M. Cassidy

Catherine M. Cassidy
Editor-in-Chief
Prevention magazine

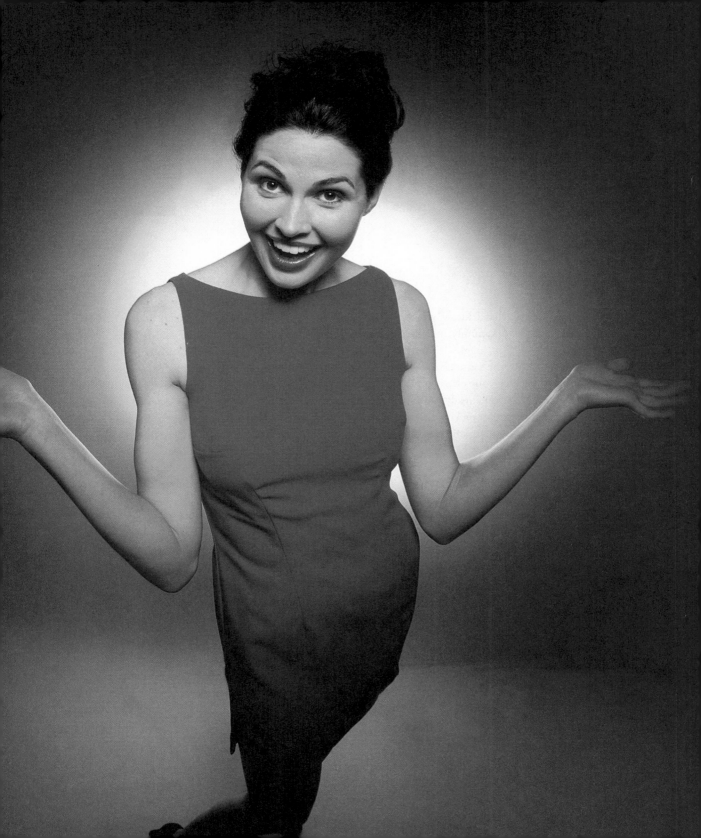

PART ONE

Drop a Dress Size in 4 Weeks!

CHAPTER 1

Lose Weight *without* Dieting!

Turn off your emotional hunger triggers, and watch extra pounds disappear

A rough Monday morning means a sundae for lunch. You just got a promotion? It's sure to be followed by a lavish dinner at your favorite eatery. And a little midday pick-me-up often comes in a candy wrapper. Do these habits sound familiar? Lots of women use food for celebration and solace. The problem is, if you rely on "food therapy" too often, you can wind up with a new problem: unwanted pounds.

Now the good news: If you're someone who deals with emotional issues by eating, you may be able to lose those unwanted pounds simply by finding better ways of coping with stress. In essence, you'll be using your mind to melt away unwanted weight! In fact, say some experts, unless you come to grips with what's going on in your head, no diet will ever work. So read on, and learn how to give emotional eating the slip, and soon you'll be slipping into smaller jeans!

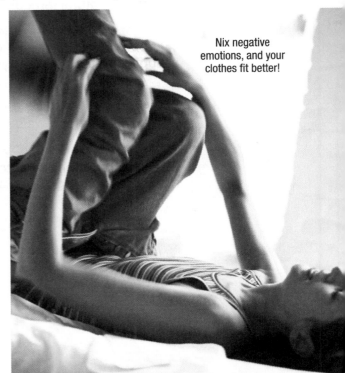

Nix negative emotions, and your clothes fit better!

When Food Equals Love

Many people struggling with their weight are what Stephen P. Gullo, PhD, a prominent weight loss expert in New York City, calls food therapists: people who use food to deal with stress and the problems of life.

"They have developed a one-word response to any and all problems: Eat!" says Dr. Gullo, author of *Thin Tastes Better* (Carol Southern Books, 1995). It's not surprising that so many people use food as a tranquilizer, says Dori Winchell, PhD, a psychologist in private practice specializing in eating disorders in Encinitas, CA. "From the time you're a baby through childhood, whenever you're unhappy, someone soothes you with a cookie. We've been pairing emotions with eating for so long that it's little wonder we know anything else." What's more, admits Dr. Winchell, food works. "Food can create soothing changes in brain chemistry, and even the simple act of chewing will increase endorphins and ease your pain."

To top it off, the stress you feel when you're upset actually makes you feel hungry and creates body fat. Stressors—everything from chronic stress from deadline pressures at work to painful baggage from your past—trigger your body to increase the production of cortisol, the hormone that encourages fat storage, particularly around the belly. Your body also pumps increased adrenaline into your bloodstream, which makes your pancreas churn out insulin. That leads to incessant hunger, explains Pamela M. Peeke, MD, MPH, assistant clinical professor of medicine at the University of Maryland School of Medicine in Baltimore and author of the bestselling book *Fight Fat After Forty* (Viking Press, 2000).

TAKE OUR QUIZ
Do You Use Food Therapy?

Just about everyone succumbs to temptation once in a while. But some women turn to the fridge for solace more often than others. How much do *you* turn to food for therapy? Here's how to tell: Rate each of the following statements from 1 to 5, with 1 being rarely true to 5 being almost always true. If it never is true, use 0.

____ There is no problem that can't be made better with chocolate.

____ I like to treat myself to a nice dinner (or other food treat) to celebrate a job well done.

____ On previous diets, I've sometimes cheated because I just felt I deserved a little treat.

____ When I'm particularly stressed or upset, I usually feel better after I've eaten something.

____ I have a favorite restaurant where friends and I usually go to celebrate or just be together.

____ I have a particular food I always crave when I'm under stress.

____ I always gain weight when I'm under pressure.

____ Whenever I've gone off a diet plan, there was something unpleasant going on in my life.

____ I always overeat when I go home to visit my parents.

____ I always overeat after a fight with my significant other.

If you scored 21 or less, you may occasionally use food for solace, but you're basically an unemployed food therapist.

If you scored 22 to 36, you are employed as a food therapist part-time.

If you scored 37 or more, you are one of the legions of people who turn to food first and foremost to treat distress. If you practice food therapy more than once in a while, this chapter is for you!

From *Thin Tastes Better* by Stephen P. Gullo, PhD. Copyright © 1995 by Stephen Gullo Food Control Center. Used by permission of Crown Publishers, a division of Random House, Inc.

You eat for relief, which, unfortunately, lasts only as long as the last bite. Then the problems you were trying to solve with food suddenly reappear. (They never went away.) And you feel like a failure: Not only didn't you solve your problems, you created a new one—right there around your waist!

To find out if you're practicing food therapy, take Dr. Gullo's quiz "Do You Use Food Therapy?" on p. 3. Then read on, and find the *right* tools to attack emotional angst. In the time it would take to forage for your favorite quick-fix food, you can take steps to break the cycle, beat stress, eliminate emotional eating, and, yes, finally drop that excess weight for good—without even trying.

Feed Your *Emotional* Hunger

Sometimes food cravings mean you want food, but often, especially for emotional eaters, they're saying you want something else: It could be creative stimulation, companionship, or more satisfaction in life. That was true for Karen Jones* of Rockville, MD, who shed 70 lb from her 210-lb frame when she identified her eating triggers as boredom, frustration, and loneliness. "I'd tried, and ultimately failed, countless diets," says Jones. "But once I understood why I was eating and started confronting those issues head-on, the weight came off without any diet at all." Not sure

*Not her real name

Short-Circuit a Binge

Bingeing will be less of an issue once you've tackled the issues behind your eating, but what can you do until that happy day arrives? Use these tips to help stop a binge in its tracks the next time you catch yourself scraping the bottom of the ice cream carton and heading for the chips. "Learning from your mistakes is an important step to long-term weight loss success," says Lee Kern, clinical director at Structure House, a weight loss center in Durham, NC. So don't beat yourself up or punish yourself by going on a starvation diet after a binge. Here's how to regain control—before you regain any pounds.

1. **Take a break.** As soon as you realize what you're doing, stop. Throw out the cookie box, brush your teeth, or chew some gum, or remind yourself that 400 calories is a lot easier to deal with than 4,000.
2. **Calm down.** Take a deep breath, and distance yourself from the incident: Clean out a closet, take a shower, or just go to bed.
3. **Renew your commitment.** Next, write down why you want to lose weight. Then forgive yourself, and get right back on your healthy eating plan. Punishing yourself will only set you up for another binge.
4. **Reflect on the reasons.** Try to figure out what triggers your binges—then reschedule your day to avoid these "dangerous" situations.
5. **Call a friend.** Talking through your experience right away provides tremendous emotional relief. See Chapter 27 for more information on how friendships can help improve your health.

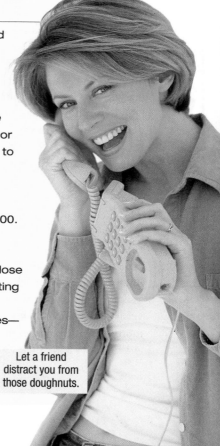

Let a friend distract you from those doughnuts.

what you're actually "hungry" for? Here's how to figure it out and "feed" it.

Shop for some stimulants. Do you eat when you're bored or need a pick-me-up? Time to make a new "grocery" list. Buy inexpensive, accessible things such as books, CDs, and tapes or DVDs—items that will provide the emotional lift you're currently seeking from food. Keep them handy, and turn to them when you're down.

Make a human connection. "For some people, food is love," says *Prevention* columnist Edward M. Hallowell, MD, psychiatry instructor at Harvard Medical School. "You may be hungry for feeling, closeness, and companionship." Or, like Karen, you eat to escape painful feelings. "Make a human connection instead," suggests Dr. Hallowell. "Call your best friend." Make sure you pick someone who makes you feel good. If you have issues with a parent or friend, calling them could lead you to finish off an entire row of cookies.

Pursue your dreams. Maybe you're hungering for a big change, such as a more satisfying career. Go for it, one small step at a time. "Take a class at a community college, or just start talking to people in that field. Moving toward goals is exhilarating," says Dr. Peeke, who saw one client drop 60 lb once she left a safe but unfulfilling job and pursued her dream of being a caterer.

Keep your hands busy. Many people eat every time there's a lull, such as during TV commercials, says eating disorders expert Sandra Haber, PhD, adjunct associate clinical professor at Adelphi University's Derner Institute in New York City. Be prepared for those lulls. "Keep manicure supplies, stacks of empty photo albums, or a cross-stitch project by the TV for something to do," she suggests. Even better, find a hobby. Or try doing

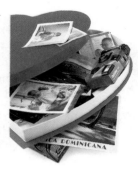

During down times, remember good times: Stick old photos in albums instead of eating chocolates.

exercises such as the ones in Chapter 7 during TV commercials or other typical snack times. When you're engrossed in something you love, you forget all about eating, especially if you're active. Falling in love with bicycling, for instance, has helped Karen Jones maintain her new 140-lb figure.

Rethink your rewards. Like most people, you probably eat to celebrate happiness too. (Don't most happy occasions involve eating?) Find new, affordable rewards such as earrings, a new nail polish, or tickets to a movie. Make a list of these healthy rewards, and post it on your fridge or snack cupboard.

Give Your Emotions a Makeover

Suppressed emotional pain can show up as excess pounds, even if that pain is from your deep past, says Dr. Winchell. Research shows that bad childhood experiences can lead to self-nurturing with food. Though you can't change the past, you *can* improve the present. Here's how.

Take action. "If dwelling on the past was a good way to burn calories, no woman would be overweight," says Dr. Peeke. "Instead of ruminating, take action." If your mother was abusive, resolve to be a better mother yourself. If certain relatives upset you, limit your time with them. And if you need help, get therapy. (See "It Worked for Me!" below for a woman who lost 40 lb after entering therapy.) When you confront your pain head-on, it gives you control of it, so you don't need food," says Karen Jones.

Speak up. "We all want harmony, but achieving true harmony doesn't mean stuffing down feelings—and food—like many women

IT WORKED FOR ME!

"I Meditated Away 40 lb!"

Meditate away 40 lb? It sounds like the promise of a shady late-night cable TV commercial, but working mother Pat Cherry, now 45, of Sacramento, is living proof that the key to trimming your waist may be right between your own ears. Today, still weighing a trim 125 lb, Pat is happy to share her weight loss secret: "My twice-daily meditations keep me slim."

Eight years ago, Pat carried 165 lb on her 5'3" frame and a host of worries in her heart. Two years later, without following any special diet or exercise plan, she had dropped 40 lb. Pat's 2-year weight loss odyssey actually began when she joined a program for emotional eaters and started seeing a therapist. She cried as she battled with long-buried issues from a painful childhood, but gradually she began to feel more in control of her life. Daily meditation helped her relax. And as her self-worth grew, her food cravings miraculously disappeared. "Every time I dealt with a new issue, I lost 3 lb," she says.

do," says Dr. Haber. "It means speaking up and letting the people in your life know how you feel. Finding that courage is empowering," she says. And it can help you deal both with the people in your life *and* food.

Rewrite history. "When was the last time you succeeded, laughed, or had a great time?" asks Dr. Winchell. "How did you feel? Rewrite your mental history books to focus on those moments, and you'll spend less time eating your sorrows away," she says. School, work, and society teach us to concentrate on our mistakes, so we can correct them. The result: We remember all the bad stuff. Every time a bad memory pops up, replace it with a good one. You'll feel better about your life.

Be good to yourself. For a day, pretend you have a cartoon bubble over your head, and catch everything you say to yourself, suggests Dr. Haber. Write it down, and read it back. Negative self-talk keeps you buried in your pain. "Keep saying you're fat and lazy, and it's little wonder that you hide away and feed yourself junk," she says. Instead, offer yourself the same encouragement you'd give to a friend. It feels artificial at first, but when you catch yourself saying something mean, stop, and make it nice."

Feed your soul. Nurturing your spiritual self is a way to heal pain and lose weight. In surveys by The Solution—a weight loss program that focuses on skills in self-nurturing and setting limits—program founder Laurel Mellin, RD, the author of a book by the same name (*The Solution,* Regan, 1998) found that the 73% of participants who develop a deeper sense of spirituality are more likely to maintain their weight loss and lose seven times as much weight as those who don't gain spiritual depth.

Do a Daily 5-Minute Meditation

Meditation instructor Jim Malloy of St. Petersburg, FL, offers this easy-to-do meditation technique that only requires you to do it once a day for 5 minutes.

1. Find a quiet, comfortable place where you won't be distracted.

2. Sit with your back straight. Place your hands in a comfortable position. Close your eyes, or allow them to rest downward, not focused on anything. Let your breathing become deep and rhythmic.

Close your eyes, and clear your mind.

3. If you like, you can call on God or a "higher power" to help you. It's okay to let your attention drift a bit, but stay relaxed.

Don't worry about doing it right. You simply want to clear your head and relax. Remain in this state for at least 5 minutes or longer, if you can spare the time. (It works even better if you give it 20 minutes, twice a day.) The benefits of regular relaxation will extend far beyond your weight loss efforts!

Church is one place to find spiritual purpose, but there are other places to look. "Try volunteering," says Dr. Peeke. "Serve food at a shelter. Help an adult learn to read. When you teach someone else, you learn to believe in yourself. You also get in touch with your human spirit."

Boost your self-worth. Do your childhood memories include kids taunting you for being fat? Don't let that define you, says Dr. Peeke. "Say, 'Okay, I have a problem with weight, but that doesn't make me a terrible person.' Focus on something you do well. Are you a good listener? When you succeed at something, your self-worth increases, and you feel able to succeed in other areas of life too."

‖ Learn to Relax

To completely conquer emotional eating, you need to trump stress, the source of anxiety and artificial food-cravings. "I was amazed to learn that all my pangs didn't mean I was really hungry," says Naomi Henderson, 58, an entrepreneur in Bethesda, MD, who found herself growing along with her new company. "I'd eat a full meal and be ravenous 45 minutes later! All my cravings were from stress." Stress-taming tricks such as beginning each day with a 20-minute blissful bath instead of a hurry-up shower helped her drop from a size 18 to a 12.

Of course, tried-and-true stress-blasters such as steamy baths and good books help douse stress for the moment. But to really give it the heave-ho, you need to stress-proof your body with lasting relaxation exercises. Two of the best: yoga and meditation.

For an easy, relaxing meditation, see "Do a Daily 5-Minute Meditation" above.

For seven easy yoga stretches you can do to de-stress throughout the day, turn to Chapter 10.

CHAPTER 2

Fill Your Plate— Lose *More* Weight!

Try this no-diet, no-work portion-control plan today!

Hate to calculate fat percentages and count calories? Great news: You don't have to! (All those numbers are enough to make your head spin!) That's why we're offering a much simpler suggestion instead: Take a good look at your plate. When you eat, you want to fill about half or more with vegetables and/or fruits and the remainder with roughly equal amounts of starch and a high-protein food. Then watch the weight come off. It's that easy!

We even had one of our own *Prevention* readers test-drive this fill-your-plate program, and she dropped pounds, got fitter, and felt better after just 2 months of following this simple strategy. Now you can too.

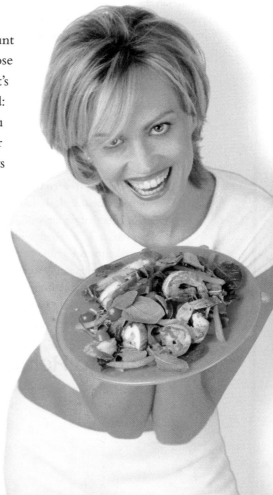

All this for lunch?
Your plate
says "Yes!"

Divide Your Plate to Lose Weight

By using your plate as a weight loss tool, you no longer have to remember confusing details about portions and servings, says Netty Levine, RD, a nutritionist at Cedars-Sinai Medical Center in Los Angeles.

"I recently worked with a client for an hour, hammering out a fabulous, detailed weight loss plan," recalls Levine. "When we finished, he looked up, and I could see it in his eyes: We'd both just wasted our time. He didn't want to remember all that information on servings and portions and food groups."

So Levine took out a fresh piece of paper and drew a big, round circle with a line through the middle. "This is your plate; fill the top half with fruits and vegetables, and divide the bottom half in two. In one quarter, put your protein, such as meat, poultry, or fish, and in the remaining quarter put your starch, such as whole grains, potatoes, or pasta," she advised.

Four months later, that client, Bill Knapp, was 28 lb lighter and loving his plate plan. "I still go to my favorite restaurants, but now I know what to order to get the right amount of food," he says.

That's the beauty of this divided-plate concept: built-in portion control. "You fill the divided plate once. If you're still hungry, have another plate of vegetables, and then you're done. It's that simple," says Levine. And with a plate half filled with vegetables, there's no room for the megacalorie, gigantic burgers and pasta "hills" notorious for contributing to the obesity epidemic.

"Everything today is supersized, and people are confused about how much they really should eat," says Nancy Vuckovic, PhD, investigator at Kaiser Permanente Center for Health Research in Portland, OR. "The overweight people coming into my office are not eating a cheeseburger, they're eating supersized meals with giant burgers, mounds of fries, and huge sodas," says Levine. The divided-plate strategy eliminates this problem, since there's simply not room for all that meat and starch when half the plate is filled with veggies and/or fruits. It brings out-of-control portions back down to size. And you're still eating enough food to feel full and satisfied.

1-MINUTE *FAT BLASTER*

Make Some Fast-Fix Veggies

If making vegetables seems like too much work, try these tricks for adding them to your diet easily.

Nothing's simpler than the salad bar!

Buy salad bar fixings. Buy prewashed and peeled baby carrots, grape tomatoes, and chopped cauliflower and broccoli from the salad bar at your supermarket. Just consider the added cost an investment in your good health!

Use precut frozen vegetables. All you have to do is steam, microwave, or lightly sauté them in olive oil with a little garlic.

Whip up a two-step salad. Chop up a ripe tomato and cucumber, dress with 2 teaspoons of olive oil and balsamic vinegar, and there you have it: a vegetable salad (which counts as two servings of veggies).

"My Stylish Clothes Fit Again!"

For Janice Williams, a typical day before using The New American Plate* was fries, fried chicken, and a biscuit for lunch; barbecued ribs and white bread for dinner. Two months later, a typical lunch was one piece of roasted chicken with peas, carrots, and rice, and pineapple for dessert.

"I've fallen in love with pineapple," she enthuses. After years of diets and weight watching, she "doesn't do scales," but she's got an even better gauge of weight loss.

"Two Sundays ago, I went to church in this smart black suit that I haven't been able to fit in for years. A woman came up to me and said, 'I know that's a size 12, so give it to me when it doesn't fit you anymore,'" Janice chuckles. She's averaging four fruits and vegetables daily, which is four times more than when she began, and she's striving for more.

*Janice was using the American Institute for Cancer Research's brochures and placemat showing The New American Plate proper plate portions. See "Dishing Out Weight Loss" on p. 12 for ordering information.

More Benefits of the Fill-Your-Plate Program

We loved this idea so much, we decided to dig a little deeper. What we found was better than we could have hoped. Not only were there other dietitians using divided-plate plans for weight loss, but also the American Institute for Cancer Research (AICR) in Washington, DC, has been harnessing the power of plates to fight cancer! In a campaign titled "The New American Plate," the AICR has released a set of free brochures as well as a placemat you can buy showing the plate portions they recommend to stave off cancer and promote weight loss (a cancer fighter in itself).

The AICR recommends portions similar to the ones described above with some slight variation. "Our rule of thumb, using a standard 9" or 10" dinner plate: Plant-based foods such as vegetables, fruits, whole grains, and beans should cover two-thirds or more of the plate. Meat, fish, poultry, or low-fat dairy should cover one-third or less of the plate," explains Melanie Polk, RD, director of nutrition education at AICR. (See "Dishing Out Weight Loss" on p. 12.)

These plate strategies fight disease because of all the fruits and vegetables they include, says James Shikany, DPH, assistant professor of medicine, division of preventive medicine, University of Alabama at Birmingham. "Studies of diet and disease indicate that the quarter of the population with the lowest intake of fruits and vegetables has double the rate of the most common cancers, such as colon, breast, and prostate," he says.

All this sounded so good to us that we decided to test-drive it ourselves. We introduced a *Prevention* reader volunteer to the AICR New American Plate plan and had her follow it for 2 months. The results were outstanding. She boosted her energy and dropped pounds simply by dividing her plate. (See "It Worked for Me!" above.)

Your Plate-Filling Cheat Sheet

There's one potential pitfall to the divided-plate concept: piling food up too high. The rule here: Go sky-high with fruits and veggies if you like; but keep the portions of starch and protein to no more than ¾" to 1" high. Or leave nothing to chance, and get the Perfect Portions Diet Dish (see p. 12); if the lid doesn't fit, your portions are too big.

No matter which plate portion variation you choose, enthusiasts insist that this method works for every meal and every food. Follow these tips whenever you eat.

Breakfast Plates

Though breakfast isn't always a meal you eat off a plate, you can still use the same portion rule when deciding how much to eat. The key is to aim for half or more of the meal to be fruits and vegetables. Here are some satisfying breakfasts to try:

Fruit-topped whole grain cereal with milk and a glass of orange juice

Vegetable-stuffed three-egg-white omelette with whole grain toast and fresh fruit or juice

Two whole grain waffles smothered in chopped fruit with a side of yogurt or milk

Fruit or juice with a small bran muffin and a glass of low-fat milk

---

DO JUST ONE THING!

Wear 9 Bracelets a Day!

Chances are that by following the fill-your-plate program in this chapter, you'll be eating about nine servings of fruits and vegetables each day. And that's great, because that's the number many experts now recommend for getting the full disease-fighting benefits of these amazing superfoods. Need a quick reminder to aim for nine servings? First, go shopping! Buy yourself nine beaded or bangle bracelets. Every morning, place all the bracelets on one wrist. Then move one bracelet to your other wrist each time you eat a fruit or veggie. Make sure all the bracelets have moved by the end of the day. It's that simple!

Here's what one fruit or veggie serving looks like:

½ cup of cut veggies or fruit
1 cup of raw, leafy greens
1 medium piece of whole fruit
¼ cup of dried fruit
¾ cup of juice

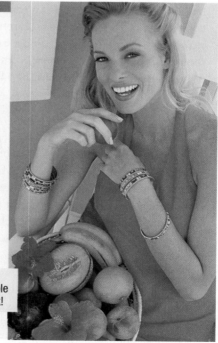

Try this fashionable diet trick!

Dishing Out Weight Loss

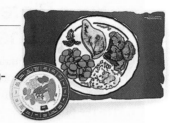

Here are some handy tools to help you stay with the plate program.

From AICR: three free brochures detailing the program, with tips, recipes, and a portion wheel. A placemat with life-size drawings of vegetables, rice, and chicken on a plate is also available. Cost: brochures and wheel are free; $2 for placemat. To order, call (800) 843-8114, or go to www.aicr.org.

Perfect Portions Diet Dish: a translucent dish (sectioned off for various types of food) that fits into a sturdy plastic base. Comes with 10 different disks that you slip between the base and the see-through plate that offer portion tips for different meals. Includes a wallet-size card of restaurant tips.

The plate is designed to provide 400- to 500-calorie meals, says co-inventor Kim Gorman, RD, a research dietitian and exercise physiologist at Akron City Hospital in Ohio. She says that the plate has helped her patients lose 20 to 50 lb over a 6-month period. Cost: $19.99. To order, call (800) 606-2468, or go to www.perfectportions.com.

The Diet Plate: a charming, earthenware dinner plate imported from the United Kingdom. Its pattern includes a measuring tape motif delineating the various sections of the plate (vegetables, starches, meats) and even a cheese square denoting ½ oz. "Salad is unlimited, and if there's not room on the plate, use a side dish," recommends inventor Kay Illingworth. Cost: $28.50. To order, go online to www.thedietplate.com, or call 011-1457-862446. (Note: This is an international call.)

Lunch Plates

As with all other meals, at least half of your lunch should be vegetables and fruits. Make sure to choose an 8" luncheon plate (measure yours if you're not sure of the size), then fill it according to our simple portion-control formula. Consider bread, tortillas, potatoes, or beans as your starch (beans serve as both starch and protein). And make a pledge to always finish your veggies or fruits first. If you have room, you can finish the rest of your meal. Here are some sample lunches you'll love:

Sandwich filled with two or three slices of lean meat, poultry, a few spoonfuls of reduced-fat tuna salad, or a veggie burger patty, with a salad, fruit salad, or vegetables

Bean-based soup (such as black bean or lentil) with a salad or side dish of vegetables or fruits

Baked potato with a cup of broccoli or other vegetable and reduced-fat cheese

Large salad topped with grilled chicken/lean beef/seafood (your protein portion should be about the size of a deck of cards) and one or two slices of whole grain bread

Burrito made from one tortilla stuffed with beans and chicken with a salad or large side dish of vegetables or fruits

Dinner Plates

You're in luck when you've got a meal comprised of distinctly different foods. But it takes some imagination to divvy up your plate when the menu calls for a casserole, stew, or other meal where the foods are combined. Just do your best to get half of the meal from fruits and veggies, and you're good to go. Here are some sample meals.

Traditional meat and potatoes. About half of the plate: salad or cooked vegetables; one-third to one-quarter of the plate: deck-of-cards-size fish, poultry, or lean meat; final quarter: rice, roll, polenta, or other starch.

Casserole or starchy mixed dish (such as lasagna or tuna noodle casserole). Make it about one-third of the plate total, no more than a cup's worth, and fill the other two-thirds with salad or vegetables.

Stir-fry. Make it three-quarters vegetables and one-quarter meat, poultry, or seafood. Fill the plate three-quarters with stir-fry and one-quarter with rice.

Pasta. Stretch 1 or 1½ cups of pasta with an equal amount or more of vegetables. Throw in a few pieces of shrimp, chicken, or soy "meat" for protein and flavor. Sprinkle Parmesan or low-fat cottage or ricotta cheese on top.

Restaurant Tips

The key here is communication with the server. Bring in a quick sketch of the ideal plate; let the waiter guide your choice. In fast-food restaurants and diners where the staff may not be helpful, order à la carte or side dishes in the proportions you want.

Inquire about portion size. If it's huge, ask the waiter for a "to-go" box, and put half of the protein and starch in the container before you start to eat. Or split the meal with your dinner partner.

Look for low-fat vegetables. Beware of foods such as the creamed spinach and roasted potatoes, which are loaded with fat. Instead, order the mixed vegetables or corn (unless it's creamed). Steamed or raw veggies are also a good choice, as long as they aren't laden with dressings or fatty sauces.

And that's really all there is to it! Just be sure to use this same rationale whenever you eat—be it at a party, a buffet brunch, or your coworker's wedding. The reason this method works when diets fail is that people finally learn to eat in a healthy way. You can include the foods you like, just not excessive amounts of them. You're eating balanced meals, and you're eating enough to feel satisfied. Even more satisfying is how good you'll look and feel.

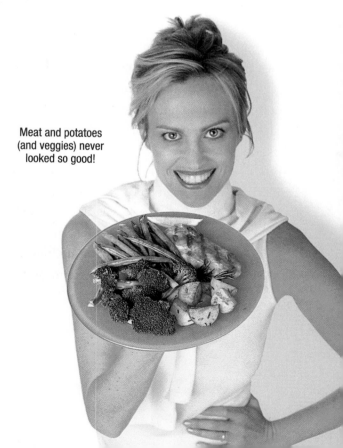

Meat and potatoes (and veggies) never looked so good!

CHAPTER 3

Turn On Your Weight Loss Hormones!

Balance out-of-whack hormones, and melt stubborn pounds forever!

If you're like most women, you view hormones as the enemy in your struggle with weight—and with good reason. Women have long believed that menstrual periods, menopause, and hysterectomies all work to keep extra pounds right where they are. So it may not surprise you that research has uncovered several bona fide links between women's hormones, hunger, and fat metabolism. Fortunately, preliminary evidence also suggests that taking advantage of your body's hormones can also *help* you to manage your weight, shape, and appetite.

What follows is a hormone-harmonizing plan, based on the latest data. Each week, you'll learn a new way to keep the levels of "snacking" hormones from inching up into the danger zone or to encourage the

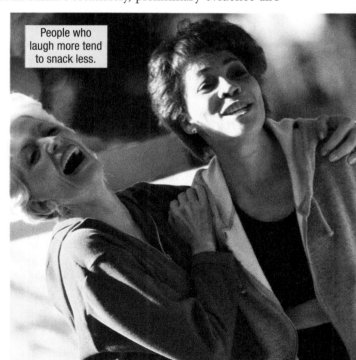

People who laugh more tend to snack less.

levels of "feel-good" hormones to rise. Work these healthy hormone habits into your regular routine, and a month from now, you just may fit into your skinny pants!

‖ Week One

Relax

If you're like many women, you've got a demanding job, a family who needs you, and a never-ending to-do list. No wonder you feel tired or depressed, anxious or irritable. Or perhaps you can't sleep (although you have no problem eating). Sex—or at least good sex—is a distant memory.

All these are hallmark symptoms of chronic stress. Stress activates the fight-or-flight response, the body's involuntary response to a threat that makes our hearts pound and our breath shorten. Chief among the hormones released during this response is the stress hormone cortisol. Cortisol automatically kicks up your appetite, prompting you not only to want to eat huge quantities but especially to want sweets and simple carbohydrates. These are foods that make insulin levels spike and then plummet, which may leave you feeling hungrier than ever and eating again, says *Prevention* advisor Pamela M. Peeke, MD, MPH, assistant clinical professor of medicine at the University of Maryland School of Medicine in Baltimore and author of *Fight Fat After Forty* (Viking Press, 2000). To help reduce stress-related hormonal cravings, experts recommend the following strategies:

Display soothing photos in your "stress zones." In the car, clip a vacation photo to your visor for a calming visual when you're stuck in traffic. In your work area, surround yourself with pictures of your children.

1-MINUTE *FAT BLASTER*

Say "No" to Fat-Free Foods

Compare labels of fat-free treats with their full-fat versions, and you're likely to find that, in many cases, the calories of fat-free foods are as high or higher. That's because sugar and other quickly digested simple carbohydrates are used to make up for the fat-based ingredients. Eat too many fat-free goodies, and your blood sugar could soar, then crash—leaving you hungry again.

Laugh. In one study conducted at Loma Linda University's Center for Neuroimmunology in California, a group of men who watched a funny video were shown to have 30% less cortisol in their blood and significantly lower levels of another stress hormone, epinephrine, during and after the tape compared with a group that sat quietly. Lighten up your commute with a cassette or CD of your favorite comedian or a humorous book on tape. Keep an eye out for funny newspaper headlines or ads. And make it a point to watch movies that make you laugh.

Get a massage. Deep-pressure massage stimulates the nerves that cause our levels of the stress hormones cortisol and epinephrine to go down, while the levels of two mood-regulating brain chemicals rise. This was true in studies of breast cancer patients conducted at the Touch Research Institute at the University of Miami School of Medicine, and of women with fibromyalgia and chronic fatigue syndrome. Both groups reported reduced anxiety and depression and improved mood and quality of life. Research also shows that folks who *give* a massage reduce their own levels of stress hormones.

Make love. The more we have sex, the more endorphins our brains release. These "neuro hormones," chemicals released in the brain during exercise and, yes, after sex, are natural painkillers and also help to alleviate anxiety.

Week Two
Get a Good Night's Rest

Besides making you cranky, one theory is that sleep loss (that is, getting less than 8 hours of sleep a night) may contribute to weight gain by dramatically disrupting the hormones that control your eating habits and your metabolism.

In one small study, researchers in the University of Chicago's department of medicine compared the hormone levels of 11 men while they got 8 hours of sleep for several nights, followed by several nights of a mere 4 hours in bed. During the sleep-debt stage, the men's ability to process glucose was impaired as much as a person with type 2 diabetes—indicating that sleep debt could lead to insulin resistance, a condition some experts think encourages obesity. In all the afternoons that followed a sleep-deprived night, the men also had consistently elevated levels of cortisol, which encourages your cells to store more fat, particularly when paired with insulin resistance. Not to mention the fact that levels of thyroid hormone (the metabolism powerhouse) were lowered during sleep deprivation.

Whether you have trouble falling asleep or staying asleep, these expert tips should help:

Get outside. The release of hormones in your brain is regulated by the nerve impulses sent by your retinas in response to light. In other words, living by the earth's natural cycle of light and darkness keeps your serotonin and cortisol at their proper levels. Getting at least 30 minutes of natural light a day helps reset your inner alarm clock, so you'll want to fall asleep at the right time, says Joyce Walsleben, PhD, director of the Sleep Disorders Center at New York University in New York City and author of *A Woman's Guide to Sleep: Guaranteed Solutions for a Good Night's Rest* (Crown Publishing Group Inc., 2000).

DO JUST ONE THING!
Stop Skipping Meals!

Do you sometimes fast most of the day, then eat just one big meal? That's a recipe for fatigue and possibly even heart attack. "Your body needs to be refueled throughout the day," explains Patty Kirk, RD, nutritionist at The Cooper Clinic in Dallas. "Eat just one meal, and you'll be dragging most of the time." And when you consume 50 g of fat at one sitting—easy to do at one big meal—your arteries lose flexibility for the next 4 hours, a period of time that one researcher has described as a "heart attack danger zone." So be sure to eat three meals a day or a series of minimeals on a regular basis.

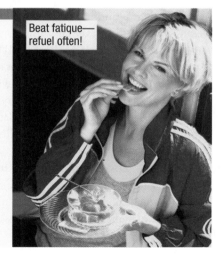
Beat fatique— refuel often!

Take a walk. In one study of more than 700 people, those who took daily walks were one-third less likely to have trouble sleeping until their normal wake-up time. Those who walked briskly slashed the risk of any sleep disorder by half. Regular exercise alleviates stress and also raises body temperature, which primes us for slumber.

Reduce or eliminate stimulants, such as caffeinated coffee, tea, soda, chocolate, and nicotine, before going to bed. Also, avoid alcohol, which is sedating but disrupts sleep.

Make your bedroom dark. Darkness stimulates the production of melatonin, a light-sensitive hormone produced by the pineal gland, which is located in the brain. Some evidence suggests that supplementing with this hormone can help remedy insomnia. (Take supplements only temporarily under the supervision of a knowledgeable medical doctor.) To manipulate this hormone naturally, invest in thick, heavy curtains, or don an eye mask.

‖ Week Three
Eat Right

A healthy diet can have a dramatically positive effect on hormone levels. The basic plan? A diet that's loaded with whole grains, fresh fruits and vegetables, and low-fat or fat-free dairy products, and that contains less red meat and processed foods.

For one thing, a high-fiber diet can help keep your blood sugar levels stable. Otherwise, foods made with refined grains (such as white bread, white pasta, and white rice) are digested quickly and speeded into the bloodstream, causing wild fluctuations in your body's levels of insulin and blood sugar and the release of the stress hormone cortisol. By contrast, beans, brown rice, and whole

Prevent the PMS Munchies

If out-of-control cravings drive you to the cookie jar every month, here's what you can do to avoid packing on extra pounds over the long haul.

First, realize that it's normal to experience food cravings around the time of your period, says *Prevention* advisor Pamela M. Peeke, MD, MPH. The menstrual cycle delivers a double whammy of two different hormone groups increasing at the same time: sex hormones (estrogen and progesterone) and stress hormones (cortisol and epinephrine). These changes drive up your appetite and prompt you to eat foods loaded with empty calories.

To minimize the munchies, here's what Dr. Peeke recommends:

Eat a little more protein, such as an egg or a cup of beans, at every meal when you have PMS to help prevent wild cravings. "Protein can give you an exquisite sense of satisfaction," says Dr. Peeke.

Get your calcium (the recommended Daily Value of 1,000 mg a day from food and supplements). Research shows that it works to reduce PMS cravings.

Exercise, no matter how bad you feel. The aerobic charge will dampen your appetite.

Excerpted from *The Hormone Connection* by Gale Maleskey, Mary Kittel, and the editors of *Prevention* (Rodale Inc., 2001). Available wherever books are sold, directly from the publisher by calling (800) 848-4735, or by visiting www.rodalestore.com.

grain cereals take much longer to digest. Thus, insulin levels rise gradually, blood sugar levels remain steady, and cortisol levels don't skyrocket.

Here are some other diet tips to help trick your weight control hormones with food.

Try "minimeals." Instead of eating three big meals a day—plus random snacks—eat five or six smaller meals spaced evenly throughout the day. Keep each meal between 250 and 350 calories. "By eating smaller yet more frequent meals, with correct proportions of proteins, fats, and carbohydrates, you may be manipulating your hormones in favor of reaching the weight you want," says Geoffrey Redmond, MD, director of the Hormone Center of New York in New York City and author of *The Good News about Women's Hormones* (Warner Books, Inc., 1995).

Make breakfast a must. It is the "single greatest factor in maintaining portion control and stable hormone levels throughout the day," says Dr. Redmond.

Begin with a protein appetizer. Eating a protein-rich food 10 minutes before a meal may prevent overeating since protein stimulates the production of the appetite-regulating hormones cholecystokinin and glucagon. Have string cheese or a very small handful of nuts before you sit down to dine.

‖ Week Four
Move That Body

Lacing up your sneakers is virtually a call to action for the hormones that reverse fat storage and curb eating. "Your muscles are loaded with insulin receptors," says Christiane Northrup, MD, author of *The Wisdom of Menopause* (Bantam Books, 2001). "The more muscle mass you have and the more heat you generate from your muscles on a regular basis, the more efficiently you'll use insulin and burn carbohydrates and body fat."

There's also strong evidence that moderate exercise—a brisk walk or a 45-minute weight training session—also triggers the release of "pleasure chemicals" known as endorphins. Finally, working up a good sweat activates the "feel-good" neurotransmitters dopamine and serotonin, which reduce the symptoms of depression. For a great exercise plan that can help speed weight loss and regulate hormone levels, turn to Part Two, starting on p. 46.

The HRT Myth

You may have heard that taking hormone replacement therapy (HRT) can cause weight gain. Not so.

Of the 875 women who participated for 3 years in a study known as the Postmenopausal Estrogen/Progestin Interventions (PEPI) trial, those who used HRT actually gained less weight than nonusers. Better yet, other studies of postmenopausal women showed that those on estrogen therapy actually *reduced* the trickiest fat storage area of all: their abdominal region.

CHAPTER 4

Safe Weight Loss Herbs That Work

Overcome common diet and exercise obstacles with these natural remedies

You already know that a healthy diet and regular exercise are the keys to a successful weight loss program, but did you know that certain herbs can help improve your chances of staying the course? Of course, you've probably *also* heard that some herbal weight loss aids aren't the safest products on the market. That's why we've come up with this handy guide to safe and effective herbal supplements that can help you pare pounds more quickly. In this chapter, you'll find information on nine herbs that can boost your willpower, keep you energized, help you feel full on fewer calories, and rev up your metabolism.

"I've recommended these botanicals in my clinical practice for the past 10 years," asserts clinical herbalist and *Prevention* advisor

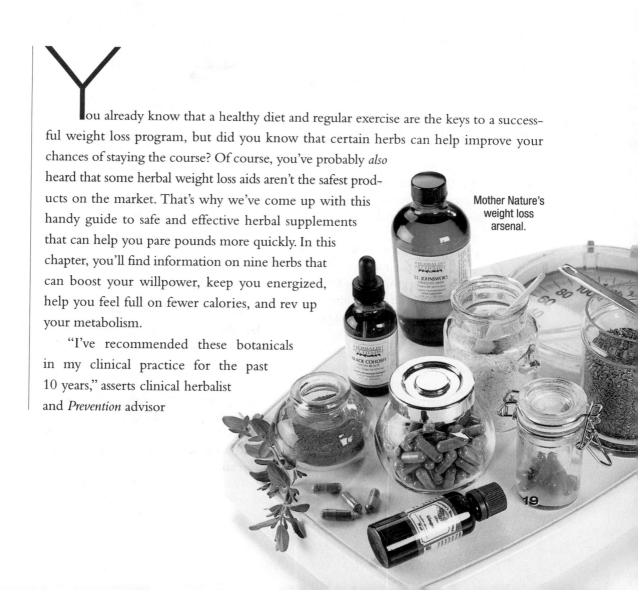

Mother Nature's weight loss arsenal.

19

Douglas Schar, DipPhyt, MCPP, MNIMH, "and I can tell you from personal observation that, when used as directed, they work." By helping you say no to supersize portions and the all-too-inviting sofa, these herbs can help you reach your weight loss goal. Here's what you need to know to put them to use.

Boost Your Willpower

Wherever you go, food is in your face. Bookstores peddle pastries; shopping malls station candy, pretzel, and ice cream stands at every turn; and you can fill 'er up at gas stations on pizza, subs, and fried chicken—not to mention all those aisles of chips and candy bars.

To lose weight, you have to resist constant temptation. And that means having nerves of steel, because frazzled nerves are a prescription for dietary disaster when the dessert cart rolls your way.

Herbal medicine offers tonics that shore up the nervous system and make it more resilient to everyday stresses. They can give you the fortitude you need to resist the vending machine when your boss has you at your wit's end. What's more, these herbs boost your mood. Just as a bad mood can trigger an eating binge, an upbeat attitude is the best defense against diving into the doughnuts at work.

Putting the herbs to work: Select the nerve tonic below that most directly addresses your needs. Start taking it a month before you begin your weight loss program, and take it regularly for best results. These herbs can be safely used for an unlimited period of time.

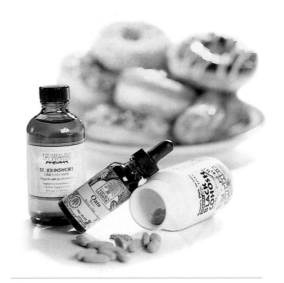

Oat straw, black cohosh, and St. John's wort can help you beat bad-mood binges.

The Binge Preventer
St. John's Wort (*Hypericum perforatum*)

Though St. John's wort is usually thought of as an herbal antidepressant, it's also a tonic that strengthens the nervous system by ensuring a steady supply of the neurotransmitters needed for proper function. It's the right choice if you tend to succumb to overeating when you're under stress.

Take one of the following three times a day:

Tincture (1:5): 1 teaspoon (5 milliliters [ml])

Tincture (1:1): 20 drops
Tableted dried herb: two 500-mg tablets
Tableted standardized extract: tablets containing the equivalent of 0.3 mg hypericin

Willpower Herb
Oat Straw *(Avena sativa)*

In the previous century, the Eclectics (holistic physicians who believed in treating the causes of illness rather than the symptoms) found that this herb helped alcoholics, smokers, and heroin addicts summon the will to "just say no" to their addiction. They also found that it helped addicts overcome symptoms of withdrawal. If you're having a hard time summoning willpower, find some oat straw.

Take one of the following three times a day:
Tincture (1:5): 1 teaspoon (5 ml)
Tincture (1:1): 20 drops

Menopause Mood Modulator
Black Cohosh *(Cimicifuga racemosa)*

Menopause-related mood swings and hot flashes make dieting a nightmare and can lead to nerve-soothing sessions with chocolate. Black cohosh is an effective weapon when hormonal mood swings threaten your weight loss efforts. Caution: Do not use black cohosh if you're taking hormone replacement therapy.

Take one of the following three times a day:
Tincture (1:5): 1 teaspoon (5 ml)
Tincture (1:1): 20 drops
Tableted dried root: two 500-mg tablets
Tableted dry extract (4:1): 250 mg
Standardized dry extract: one tablet containing 1 mg 27-deoxyacteine

‖ Get More Energy

You know how important it is to increase your activity level to lose weight. Not only does exercise help the weight come off faster—it also makes you feel and look better in the long run. The problem is having the energy to become active. When you're pooped, you'll probably pass on the push-ups and opt for channel surfing instead. Exhaustion also makes it easier to substitute fast, fatty foods for healthy ones. Herbal remedies known as adaptogens can help, because they increase stamina and endurance and give you the boost you need to get to the gym or outside for a walk. And once you're there, adaptogens will help energize your exercise session.

Putting the herbs to work: The following two herbs work immediately and do not need to be taken for long periods of time to be effective. Take a dose half an hour before hitting the gym or the walking path.

More Herb Info

You can find more information on herbs in our Healing Herbs database on our Web site. You'll also find links to informative herb-related features from past issues of *Prevention* magazine. Just go to www.prevention.com/news.

DO JUST ONE THING!

Avoid Dangerous Herbs

With some herbal weight loss aids, the claims usually sound too good to be true, which often means that they are. The following herbal weight loss products often contain dangerous, counterproductive, or useless ingredients. So save your money—and your health.

Herbal Laxatives

Laxative herbs are frequently added to diet products because they empty the bowel and temporarily make the stomach look flatter. But they're potentially dangerous. They contain anthraquinones, compounds that stimulate the bowel to evacuate its contents. Many experts believe that, with regular use, these herbs can damage the nerves that serve the bowel, leading to chronic constipation.

Avoid diet products containing aloe, buckthorn, cascara sagrada, rhubarb, senna, or yellow dock.

Herbal Stimulants

When you reduce your calorie intake, you sometimes feel tired and sluggish. To combat this, some manufacturers add herbal "speed" to diet products. This causes a stimulant high, which is followed by a stimulant low. In fact, you'll feel lower than you did before you took the stimulant and could set yourself up for a comfort-eating session. In addition, if you have heart disease, kidney problems, or high blood pressure, or if you take certain medications for depression or anxiety, these herbs can be downright dangerous.

Avoid products containing ephedra (ma huang), guarana, betel, mate, cola, or caffeine.

Multiherb Products

These are the "kitchen sink" supplements, products that contain as many as 20 herbs in a tablet or capsule. It's hard enough to get an active dose of one herb into a single tablet or capsule, much less 20 active doses of 20 different herbs. Bottom line: They just don't work.

Avoid diet products containing many different herbs.

Herbal Diuretics

When you urinate, you lose water weight. That's the lame justification behind adding herbal diuretics to weight loss products. Though generally harmless (unless you suffer from kidney disease), these products won't help you lose an ounce of fat.

Avoid diet supplements containing corn silk, buchu, dandelion tops, or couch grass.

The Energizer
Cordyceps (Cordyceps sinensis)

Cordyceps is an ancient Chinese remedy famous for increasing stamina and well-being. Once an extremely rare and costly herb, contemporary production techniques have made this mushroom more affordable. Bodybuilders use it to power up workout sessions, and endurance athletes use it to keep themselves going longer. With this herb, you may have to remind yourself to get *off* the treadmill!

Take one dose half an hour before exercise:

Powdered cordyceps: one 250-mg capsule

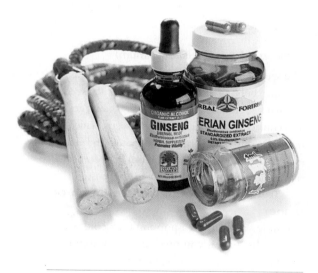

Having trouble getting motivated
to work out? Cordyceps
or Siberian ginseng
can help you get moving.

The Endurance Herb
Siberian Ginseng
(Eleutherococcus senticosus)

Long used in Asia, Siberian ginseng has been found to increase animals' ability to work and to also increase human stamina. In fact, the Russian cosmonauts used it on the job to counter the fatigue associated with long hours and lack of sleep. Many studies have shown that this herb increases the capacity to do work—in your case, at the gym.

Take one of the following half an hour before exercise:

Tincture (1:5): 1 teaspoon (5 ml)
Tincture (1:1): 20 drops
Tableted dried bark: four 500-mg tablets
Tableted standardized extract: One 100-mg tablet standardized to contain 1% or more Eleutheroside E

Feel Full on Fewer Calories

Once you begin choosing sensibly sized portions, you may discover a gnawing, empty feeling that can lead to unhealthy snacking. Though your stomach will eventually adjust to smaller portions, you may not last long enough to find that out.

Here again, herbs can help—in this case, fiber-rich, calorie-poor herbs. They fill up your stomach without any calories so that when you actually sit down to eat, you eat less. Or if you don't feel full after eating a sensible meal, a teaspoon of herbal fiber can help you feel satisfied.

Putting the herbs to work: Take a dose of either of these herbs half an hour before

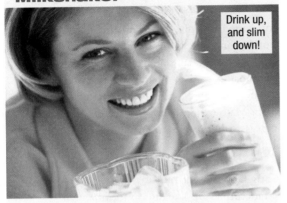

1-MINUTE *FAT BLASTER*

Make a Weight Loss Milkshake!

Drink up, and slim down!

Research has shown that the mineral calcium—found in low-fat and fat-free dairy products such as milk and cheese—acts like a key in fat cells. When calcium levels dip too low, it "turns on" the genes that lead to fat production. What's more, decreasing calcium suppresses the system that breaks down fat. To help keep your calcium level where it belongs, try this delicious recipe for meeting 40% of your daily calcium needs!

CALCIUM-RICH TROPICAL SMOOTHIE

1	c low-fat plain yogurt
1	c mango cubes
1	sm banana, sliced
½	c pineapple chunks
¼	c nonfat dry milk
1	Tbsp lime juice

In a blender, combine all ingredients. Blend until smooth.

Makes 3 cups

Per 1½-cup serving: 230 cal, 10 g pro, 45 g carb, 3 g fat, 9 mg chol, 3 g fiber, 129 mg sodium

eating. Note: For some people, these herbs may have a laxative effect. In that case, reduce your dose slightly.

The Tummy Fillers

Psyllium seed *(Plantago psyllium)*

The seed of the Indian plantain is surrounded with a coat of almost pure fiber. When this fiber comes in contact with water, it swells to four times its original size. The seed has the added benefit of reducing cholesterol levels while giving you that pleasant full sensation.

Take half an hour before lunch or dinner:

Psyllium seeds: 1 teaspoon in 8 oz cold water (If this makes you feel uncomfortably full, reduce the dose to ½ teaspoon.)

Flaxseed *(Linum usitatissimum)*

The seed of the flax plant has long been used as a soothing bulking agent. Like psyllium, flaxseed is covered with mucilage, which swells when it comes into contact with water. Use whole seeds, which go through your body largely undigested and unabsorbed. Ground flaxseed, which can be absorbed, is rich in calories and thus defeats the purpose.

Take half an hour before lunch or dinner:

Whole flaxseed: 1 teaspoon in 8 oz cold water (If this makes you feel uncomfortably full, reduce the dose to ½ teaspoon.)

Speed Up Your Metabolism

Some people are blessed with fast metabolisms. Others aren't. Fast burners regularly risk life and limb by saying things such as "I can eat all day long and never gain weight" to people who gain weight just looking at a piece of cake. As you get older and lose muscle, your metabolism slows even more. If your metabolism is sluggish, taking herbal medicine in addition to strength training may help. Experts believe that certain herbs (called thermogenic agents) activate all the cells in the body and make you burn calories more rapidly.

Putting the herbs to work: Take thermogenic herbs three times a day with meals. It's not hard to figure out if they're working; you should feel warmer 10 minutes after taking them. Some people find ginger to be more effective, while others prefer cayenne. Experiment to find out which works best for you.

The Fire-You-Up Herb
Cayenne *(Capsicum minima)*

The most famous thermogenic herb is undoubtedly mouth-burning red pepper. Eating red pepper results in more than just a hot mouth: It makes you sweat and warms your fingers and toes. Red pepper also jump-starts your circulation and gets your blood rushing all over the place.

Take one of the following three times a day:

Tincture (1:5): 10 drops

Tincture (1:1): 2 drops

Powdered cayenne pepper: ¼ teaspoon mixed with a glass of water

Tableted cayenne pepper: one 250-mg tablet

The Body Warmer
Ginger *(Zingiber officinale)*

Ginger was once consumed in huge quantities in Britain, not because of its taste but because it

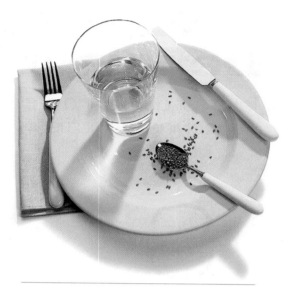

Herbal fiber
before a meal can
help curb
your appetite.

helped people survive the cold, damp climate. This made the lack of central heating a little more bearable.

Take one of the following three times a day:

Tincture (1:5): 1 teaspoon (5 ml)

Tincture (1:1): 20 drops

Root tablets: two 500-mg tablets

Powdered dried root: ½ teaspoon in a cup of boiling water

Fresh root: 1 teaspoon grated into a cup of boiling water

CHAPTER 5

Is Your Multivitamin Deficient?

Take our quiz to find out if your multivitamin is supplying the nutrients your diet lacks

So you're eating healthier now, thanks to Chapter 2, but do you still need to take a daily multivitamin supplement? Experts say yes. It's easy to fall short on a few key nutrients each day, even if you're trying your best to eat right.

"I advise everyone I counsel to take a daily moderate multi, containing about 100% of the Daily Value (DV) for most vitamins and minerals," says Colleen Pierre, RD, a registered dietitian in private practice and a frequent contributor to *Prevention*. "Although a multi is no substitute for a good diet, I believe it's sensible nutrition insurance."

The next question, though, is which multivitamin is right for you? Taking the *wrong* one can actually compromise your health. To help you learn what to look for when choosing

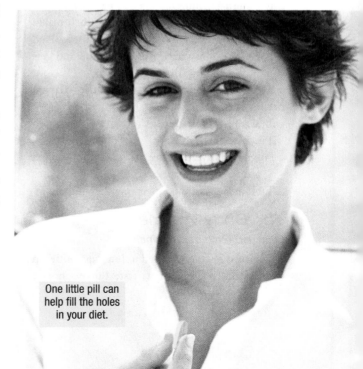

One little pill can help fill the holes in your diet.

a multivitamin (or to figure out whether or not the one you already are taking makes the grade), take the following quiz today, and start taking the right multivitamin tomorrow. (Note: Some questions have more than one right answer.)

1. For your multi to work properly, it must

 A. Disintegrate quickly

 B. Dissolve completely

 C. Be timed-release

 D. All of the above

Answer: A and B, disintegrate quickly and dissolve completely

Did you answer C, timed-release? Although that certainly sounds like a great idea, drug studies suggest that timed-release supplements might actually shortchange you on folic acid, a vitamin critical to preventing birth defects and possibly important for reducing heart disease and colon cancer. "Folic acid is absorbed high in the small intestine, just after it leaves your stomach," says Stephen Hoag, PhD, of the University of Maryland School of Pharmacy in Baltimore. That means that folic acid that's released later has missed its window of opportunity and won't be absorbed.

A and B are correct. In order for that pill you're swallowing to pass through your intestinal walls and get into your bloodstream, your stomach churns away, causing the pill to fall apart in small pieces. That disintegration allows the nutrients to dissolve in your stomach acids and get absorbed in your small intestine.

1-MINUTE *HEALTH BOOSTER*

Do the Vinegar Test

To see if your multi disintegrates quickly, drop it into ½ cup vinegar. Stir gently every now and then. In 20 minutes, your vitamin should be completely separated into tiny pieces. If not, choose another brand.

2. If you're a woman over 50, how much iron should your multi have?

 A. 0% of the DV

 B. 50% of the DV

 C. 100% of the DV

 D. 150% of the DV

Answer: A, 0% of the DV or, at the most, B, 50% of the DV

Iron is essential for red blood cell formation. But once a woman stops menstruating and losing blood each month, she normally loses very little iron and gets what she needs from her diet.

Taking in too much iron can cause constipation and other gastrointestinal problems and might cause oxidation of LDL cholesterol, increasing heart disease risks. Also, about 1 in 300 people of Northern European descent carries a gene that triggers excessive iron accumulation and can lead to liver, heart, and pancreas damage.

3. The type of copper in your multi should not be

 A. Copper sulfate

 B. Cupric sulfate

 C. Copper oxide

 D. Copper gluconate

Answer: C, copper oxide

You need a multi that disintegrates quickly and dissolves completely, making it easier for your body to absorb its nutrients.

Copper and cupric mean the same thing, and you can find a variety of combinations—such as copper sulfate, copper gluconate, copper amino acid chelate, copper glycinate chelate, and copper clycinate amino acid chelate—that work just fine. But copper oxide (or cupric oxide) is the densest form packed in a pill, and your body absorbs very little of it.

Research suggests that many people aren't getting enough dietary copper, which is needed for healthy immune systems and joints, red blood cells, and heart function. To make matters worse, zinc and copper are absorbed through similar mechanisms, so if you take a supplement packed with well-absorbed zinc and poorly absorbed copper, you can aggravate a copper deficiency, possibly weakening your immune system.

Don't worry about the other oxides in your multi, such as magnesium or zinc. They're absorbed just fine. Copper oxide is the exception.

4. If you're a woman of childbearing age, it is critical that your multi has

    A. 100% DV for vitamin A

    B. 100% DV for calcium

    C. 100% DV for iron

    D. 100% DV for folic acid

Answer: D, 100% DV for folic acid

This one is official: The Institute of Medicine, Centers for Disease Control and Prevention, and the March of Dimes all agree that any woman who could become pregnant should get 400 micrograms (mcg) of folic acid daily—*before* she becomes pregnant. And they say she should get it from a supplement or fortified food (because the synthetic form is much better absorbed) along with another 400 mcg from folate-rich foods such as OJ, broccoli, asparagus, and legumes. Studies have found that this amount can prevent neural tube birth defects, which happen in the first month after conception.

5. If you're a woman over 50, make especially sure that your multi has

    A. 100% DV for thiamin

    B. 100% DV for vitamin B_{12}

    C. 100% DV for vitamin C

    D. 100% DV for vitamin D

Answer: B and D, 100% DV for vitamins B_{12} and D

After age 50, the rate at which your stomach makes hydrochloric acid (which is needed to digest protein and release the attached vitamin B_{12}) slows down in about 10 to 30% of us. That's enough so that, on paper, your diet may look like you're getting lots of B_{12} from meat, but your digestion isn't delivering what you need. Over time, that can lead to vitamin B_{12} deficiency, causing neurological problems that often show up first as memory loss and depression. The Institute of

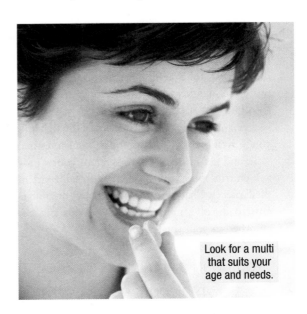

Look for a multi that suits your age and needs.

Give Your Multi a Checkup

An independent testing agency, ConsumerLab.com, recently evaluated 27 multivitamins to check disintegration, lead contamination, and folic acid, calcium, and vitamin A content. One-third of the pills tested failed and remain nameless, including one prenatal vitamin that delivered only 75% of the folic acid it promised. But for $5.25, you can get the list of those that passed. And $15.95 buys you a year's subscription to all their tests. Go to consumerlab.com/subscribe.asp, and have your credit card ready.

Medicine now advises adults over 50 to get the Recommended Dietary Allowance (RDA) of vitamin B_{12} from a supplement or fortified food.

Then there's your skin. The skin cells of 80-year-olds don't have the same capacity to synthesize vitamin D from sunlight as do those of children, so get your vitamin D from a multi. Between 51 and 70, you need 100% of the DV for vitamin D, or 400 IU. After age 70, you need 150% of the DV, which you probably won't find in a multivitamin.

Look for a separate D supplement or calcium supplement that will supply you with the extra 200 IU, but consult your doctor to make sure you're not getting too much. Vitamin D can be toxic when consumed in high doses.

6. True or false: If you're taking a prescription prenatal vitamin, you can assume it's complete with all the nutrients you need.
Answer: Amazingly enough, false

All prescription prenatals are not alike, nor are they as complete as your "regular" multivitamin, as *Prevention* Fitness Editor Michele Stanten found out when she was pregnant. The second time she had her prescription filled, she asked the pharmacist for the nutrient breakdown. The big surprise? Except for iron, there were no other minerals present, including zinc, which is needed in higher amounts during pregnancy for the fetus's growth and development.

"Any supplement designed for pregnant women should contain zinc," says Myron Winick, MD, professor emeritus of nutrition at Columbia University College of Physicians and Surgeons in New York City. Also of concern in a prenatal vitamin are the B-complex vitamins (such as B_6, B_{12}, and folic acid) that are critical for brain, nerve, and spinal cord development, and iron for blood and tissue development. So check out the multivitamin that your obstetrician prescribes to be sure it's well balanced.

Getting enough vitamin A (5,000 IU) early in pregnancy is critical for baby's development. But too much (more than 10,000 IU) of what's called "preformed vitamin A" can lead to birth defects.

To avoid exceeding the limit, add up the IUs of preformed A in any supplement you use, plus what's in any fortified foods (often including milk, cheese, and margarine). To ferret out preformed A, check ingredients lists for vitamin A palmitate, vitamin A acetate, vitamin A esters, retinal acetate, or retinal palmitate. They all count toward reaching the Safe Upper Limit of 10,000 IU.

Don't worry about getting too much A in the form of beta-carotene. Your body eliminates what you don't need.

How to Pick a Perfect Multi

Does your multivitamin measure up? Check the following chart to find out! A good multi will have close to 100% of the Daily Value (DV) for most vitamins and minerals—with important exceptions. Some people actually need more or less than the DV for certain nutrients; we list those exceptions in red. And don't expect to find a multi with 100% of the DV for everything. No multi has that much calcium, magnesium, or potassium, so in the chart we suggest how much you *should* look for.

Tempted to take higher levels? With exceptions noted below, *Prevention* does not recommend this practice. But if you do take more than the DV for any nutrient, we've also listed the Safe Upper Limit. Always stay under this level to avoid harmful or unpleasant side effects.

Vitamin/Mineral	Why It's Important	100% Daily Value	Safe Upper Limit
Vitamin A	Needed for healthy eyes and skin	5,000 IU	10,000 IU
Vitamin B_6	Used in making antibodies that fight infection	2 mg	100 mg
Vitamin B_{12}	Keeps nerves healthy	6 mcg	3,000 mcg
Vitamin C	Helps keep immune system strong (Consider taking 100 to 500 mg extra.)	60 mg* *Smokers: You need about 200% of the DV, or 120 mg, but you should really stop smoking.*	2,000 mg
Vitamin D	Makes it possible for you to absorb calcium from your food	400 IU *Over age70: Take an extra 200 IU in a separate supplement.*	2,000 IU
Vitamin E	Squelches free radicals that foster heart disease	30 IU**	1,500 IU natural 1,100 IU synthetic
Vitamin K	Essential for your blood to clot	80 micrograms (mcg)	30,000 mcg
Chromium	Works with insulin to help your body use blood sugar	120 mcg	1,000 mcg
Copper	Needed for healthy blood vessels and immune system	2 mg (not as copper oxide or cupric oxide)	10 mg

Vitamin/Mineral	Why It's Important	100% Daily Value	Safe Upper Limit
Folic acid	Critical for making perfect DNA in new cells	400 mcg	1,000 mcg
Iodine	Part of a thyroid hormone that regulates rate of energy burn	150 mcg	1,100 mcg
Iron	The part of red blood cells that carries oxygen to your body	18 mg *Postmenopausal women (and all men): 0–8mg*	45 mg
Niacin	Helps your body use sugars and fats	20 mg	35 mg (unless by prescription)
Riboflavin	Needed for energy production in all your cells	1.7 mg	200 mg
Selenium	Helps knock out free radicals that may cause cancer	70 mcg	400 mcg
Thiamin	Helps turn carbohydrates into energy	1.5 mg	50 mg
Zinc	Important for a strong immune system and wound healing	15 mg	40 mg

100% Not Available in Single Multis		What to Look For	Safe Upper Limit
Calcium	Helps make strong bones; fights high blood pressure	About 100 mg***	2,500 mg
Magnesium	For strong bones, healthy nerves and muscles	About 100 mg	350 mg
Potassium	Helps fight high blood pressure	About 40 mg	99 mg (unless by prescription)

*Consider taking 100 to 500 mg vitamin C. Some multis contain extra C, or you may need a separate supplement.

**Consider taking 100 to 400 IU vitamin E. Some multis contain extra E, or you may need a separate supplement. If you take coumadin or aspirin, consult your doctor first.

***Consider taking 500 mg calcium as a separate supplement up to age 50. Over 50, consider taking 700 mg separately—but not more than 500 mg at a time for best absorption.

CHAPTER 6

Sneak More Veggies into Dinnertime!

9 easy, family-friendly recipes, each with a healthy helping of waist-slimming vegetables

Whether your love affair with veggies began long ago or just after you learned of their waist-slimming powers in Chapter 2, it never hurts to have a few new ways to slip them into your daily meal plan. After all, there are only so many spinach salads and side dishes of green beans that one person can stand! That's why we gathered together some of the best veggie-rich main-dish recipes around—everything from Cal-Mex Tostadas to Roasted Eggplant Italian to Sweet Potato Stew! These entrees are so delicious and "mainstream" that your family will love them—and they're so healthy that you won't feel an ounce of guilt eating them yourself. (We even found fruity desserts for you to indulge in! See p. 36.)

Bon appétit!

Shop the produce aisles for tonight's meal!

‖ Cal-Mex Tostadas

Forget about those fatty taco salads you order at restaurants! With this waist-slimming Cal-Mex meal, you'll get all that flavor, less fat, and a heaping helping of veggies *and* fruit. Health bonus: This dish is packed with heart-healthy folate and fiber, as well as the antioxidant vitamin C, found in both the oranges and the salsa.

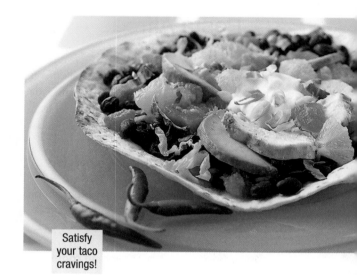

Satisfy your taco cravings!

1¼ lb boneless, skinless chicken breasts
1   c low-sodium salsa
4   med navel oranges (about ½ lb each)
2   cans (15 oz each) low-sodium black beans, rinsed and drained
4   lg fat-free flour tortillas
1   bag (8 oz) prewashed shredded lettuce
**   Fat-free sour cream, sliced avocados, sliced scallions (garnish, optional)**

1. In a resealable plastic bag, mix the chicken with ½ cup of the salsa and the juice of 1½ of the oranges. Seal the bag, and marinate in the refrigerator for 20 to 60 minutes.

2. In a 1-quart microwaveable dish with a lid, lightly mash the beans with the remaining ½ cup salsa and the juice of ½ of an orange. Microwave, covered, on high for 4 to 5 minutes, stirring halfway through the cooking time. Set aside. While the beans are cooking, peel and slice the remaining 2 oranges into ¼" thick triangles, and set aside.

3. Transfer the chicken and marinade to a medium nonstick skillet. Bring to a simmer over medium heat (about 4 minutes), then cover, and cook for 7 minutes. Turn the breasts over, and cook, covered, for an additional 7 to 8 minutes, or until the center of the meat is opaque. Remove the chicken to a platter, but leave the marinade in the pan. Slice the chicken into ¼" pieces. Cover, and set aside.

4. Meanwhile, cook the marinade, uncovered, over high heat for 5 to 6 minutes, until thickened. Remove from the heat, and set aside.

5. While the marinade is cooking, preheat the oven to 450°F. Place the tortillas directly on the rack in the center of the oven, and toast until crisp and lightly browned, about 4 to 5 minutes. Remove the tortillas from the oven, and put one on each of four dinner plates.

6. Spoon equal amounts of the bean mixture and chicken into the center of each tortilla. Surround with shredded lettuce and orange triangles. Drizzle the chicken on each plate with 1 tablespoon of the marinade. Garnish with sour cream, avocados, and scallions, if desired.

Makes 4 servings
Per serving: 514 cal, 50 g pro, 72 g carb, 6 g fat, 1 g sat. fat, 82 mg chol, 21 g fiber, 817 mg sodium

Pasta Alfredo Primavera

This basil-flavored pasta dish offers three different kinds of low-calorie veggies in a creamy sauce that's sure to satisfy the gourmet in you. Health bonus: This dish is rich in calcium, potassium, and vitamin A.

12	oz rotini or other medium-size dry pasta
1	bag (16 oz) fresh prewashed broccoli, baby carrots, and cauliflower florets, cut into bite-size pieces (about 4 c)
1	c fat-free sour cream
¼	c fat-free cream cheese, at room temperature
2	Tbsp dried basil
⅔	c grated Parmesan cheese

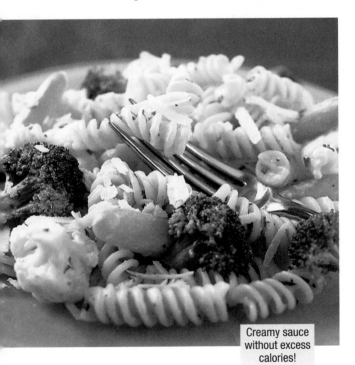

Creamy sauce without excess calories!

1. Cook the pasta per package directions. Do not add salt or oil.
2. During the last 5 minutes of cooking time, add the vegetables, and cook until they are tender.
3. Drain the pasta and vegetables well in a colander, and place them in a large bowl.
4. Place the sour cream, cream cheese, and basil in a small saucepan over medium-low heat, and mix, whisking constantly, until heated through but not bubbling.
5. Fold the sauce into the hot pasta and vegetables, then fold in the Parmesan.

Makes 4 servings
Per serving: 473 cal, 25 g pro, 77 g carb, 7 g fat, 3 g sat. fat, 14 mg chol, 5 g fiber, 462 mg sodium

Stuffed Flank Steak Spirals

Here, we paired the leanest cuts of beef with a sun-dried tomato and corn filling. Be sure to fill half your plate with a side dish of veggies when you serve this meaty meal! Health bonus: Steak is a good source of iron.

¾	c dry-packed sun-dried tomato halves
1	flank steak (about 1½ lb), trimmed
2	Tbsp balsamic vinegar
1	lg clove garlic, crushed
¼	tsp ground black pepper
¾	c frozen corn
3	lg scallions, sliced
⅓	c grated Parmesan cheese
1	egg or 2 egg whites
3	Tbsp toasted pine nuts
1	Tbsp chopped fresh oregano
⅔	c dried bread crumbs
½	tsp salt

1. Place the tomatoes in a small bowl, and cover with boiling water. Let stand for at least 20 minutes, or until softened.
2. Meanwhile, pound the steak between sheets of plastic wrap to about ¼" thickness.
3. In a small bowl, combine the vinegar, garlic, and pepper. Brush the mixture on both sides of the steak, then place the steak in a large, shallow baking dish. Cover with plastic wrap, and marinate in the refrigerator for 30 to 60 minutes.
4. Preheat the oven to 400°F. Drain and chop the tomatoes. In a medium bowl, combine the tomatoes, corn, scallions, Parmesan, egg, pine nuts, and oregano. Stir in the bread crumbs.
5. Place the steak on a large cutting board or clean surface, and sprinkle with the salt. Spread the filling evenly over the top, leaving a 1" border on the long side. Roll up from the long side, shaping the steak into a log.
6. Cut four or five 12" pieces of kitchen twine. Starting ¾" from one end, tie the meat at equally spaced intervals. Return the meat to the dish.
7. Bake for 40 to 45 minutes, or until a thermometer inserted in the center of the steak registers 145°F (medium-rare). Let stand for 10 minutes. Remove the strings, and serve.

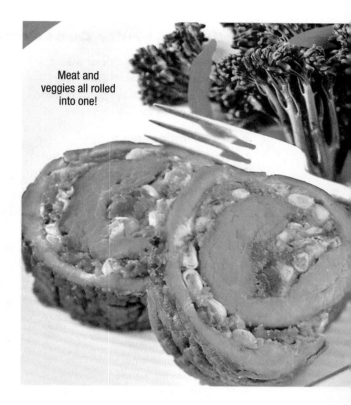

Meat and veggies all rolled into one!

Makes 7 servings
Per serving: 303 cal, 25 g pro, 17 g carb, 15 g fat, 6 g sat. fat, 85 mg chol, 1 g fiber, 397 mg sodium

DO JUST ONE THING!

Stick to Your Grocery List

You don't have to eat carrot sticks and swear off cheesecake to see permanent changes in your waistline. Out of the 7,000 participants in the Lean Habits Study—a 3-year diet project in Germany that will help determine what factors cause people to maintain weight—those who've trimmed at least 5% of their body weight and kept it off more than a year share some practical and even enjoyable habits. Among them: using a shopping list to avoid fattening impulse buys. They also peruse the produce section, check labels, and generally eat a nutritious diet.

Delicious, Fruity Desserts!

These tempting after-dinner treats will satisfy your craving for something sweet—and give you an extra helping of fruits too!

APPLESAUCE COBBLER

Not a spoonful of sugar is used in this fruit-filled, crumbly dessert—it gets all its sweetness from fresh apples. Health bonus: Apples are a top source of the antioxidant quercetin, which may help fight cancer.

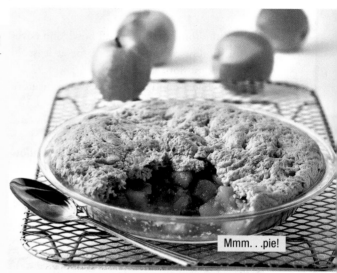

Mmm. . .pie!

8	firm, crisp cooking apples (3 lb), cored and cut into chunks (use a combination of Fuji, McIntosh, Golden Delicious, Granny Smith, and Jonathan)
½	c unsweetened apple cider
1	Tbsp lemon juice
1	stick cinnamon
½	c golden raisins
½	tsp ground nutmeg
½	c plus 2 Tbsp all-purpose flour
½	c whole wheat pastry flour
1½	tsp baking powder
½	tsp salt
¼	tsp ground cinnamon
2	Tbsp melted butter
¼	c apple juice concentrate, partially thawed
¼	c low-fat plain yogurt

1. Place the apple chunks, cider, lemon juice, and cinnamon stick in a large saucepan. Cover, and cook over medium heat, stirring occasionally, until the mixture begins to bubble. Reduce the heat to low, and cook for about 20 minutes, or until the apples are very tender.

2. Remove the pan from the heat, discard the cinnamon stick, and stir in the raisins and nutmeg. Spoon the applesauce into a 9" pie pan or shallow baking dish. (The apple mixture can be made a day ahead.)

3. Heat the oven to 400°F. In a medium bowl, stir together the flours, baking powder, salt, and cinnamon. In a small bowl, combine the butter, apple juice, and yogurt. Pour the wet mixture into the dry, and blend gently with a fork for about 30 seconds. Remove to a floured surface, and knead for about 30 seconds.

4. With floured fingertips, press and spread the dough over the applesauce, making the dough surface as even as possible. Reduce the oven temperature to 375°F, and bake for 20 to 25 minutes, or until the cobbler is golden brown. Serve warm or at room temperature.

Makes 4 servings

Per serving: 286 cal, 4 g pro, 59 g carb, 5 g fat, 3 g sat. fat, 11 mg chol, 5 g fiber, 310 mg sodium

ALL-PURPOSE BLUEBERRY SAUCE

Use this antioxidant-rich sweet topping to spruce up fat-free frozen yogurt, cornbread, or any other "boring" finale.

1	pt fresh or frozen blueberries
¼	c dry red wine
1	Tbsp orange juice

1. In a medium saucepan, combine the blueberries, wine, and juice. Bring to a boil over medium-high heat, stirring constantly. Boil for 1 minute.

2. Reduce heat to low, cover, and simmer, stirring frequently, for 5 minutes, or until the blueberries are tender and the sauce is thick. Allow the sauce to cool, and serve warm, or refrigerate it until ready to use.

Makes 1 serving

Per serving: (¼ c) 25 cal, 0 g pro, 5 g carb, 0 g fat, 0 g sat. fat, 0 mg chol, 1 g fiber, 0 mg sodium

GRANOLA-BERRY PARFAIT

You can eat this luscious layered treat for breakfast, dessert, or a snack. Feel free to use extra fruit in each serving, and substitute whatever fresh berries or fruits are in season. Health bonus: The granola provides both fiber and antioxidants.

3	c old-fashioned rolled oats
2	oz (about ½ c) slivered almonds
¼	c wheat germ
2	Tbsp shelled sunflower seeds, unsalted
1	Tbsp ground cinnamon
5	Tbsp honey
32	fl oz low-fat maple vanilla or vanilla yogurt
4	c fresh raspberries (or blueberries or sliced strawberries)

1. Preheat the oven to 325°F.

2. In a medium bowl, thoroughly mix together the oats, almonds, wheat germ, sunflower seeds, and cinnamon. Continue to stir while drizzling the honey into the mixture until thoroughly combined.

3. Spread the granola mixture evenly onto a baking sheet. Bake for 30 minutes, or until golden brown, stirring occasionally during baking.

4. Remove the granola from the oven. Let it cool to room temperature before preparing the parfaits.

5. To serve, layer the granola with the yogurt and berries in a parfait or other large beverage glass.

Makes 8 parfaits with ½ cup granola, ½ cup yogurt, and ½ cup fruit each

Note: Granola can be prepared ahead of time and stored in an airtight container for several days.

Per serving: 360 cal, 14 g pro, 57 g carb, 9 g fat, 2 g sat. fat, 0 mg chol, 4 g fiber, 88 mg sodium

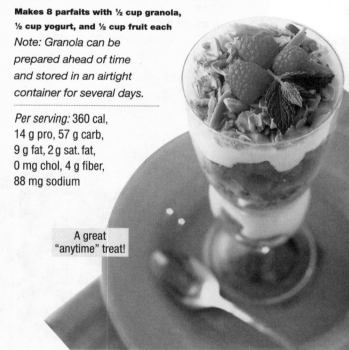

A great "anytime" treat!

Sausage and Chickpea Stew

This high-fiber stew is a delicious way to get lots of vegetables into one dish. Serve it with a spinach side salad for more vegetables (and vitamins!). Health bonus: This hearty meal offers a healthy dose of disease-fighting antioxidants.

¾	lb spicy sausage (such as chorizo or hot Italian), cut into ½" pieces
2	tsp olive oil
2	onions, chopped
1	red bell pepper, chopped
1	green bell pepper, chopped
3	cloves garlic, minced
1	tsp dried oregano
1	tsp herbes de Provence or dried thyme
1	tsp paprika
2	cans (15 oz each) diced tomatoes
1	can (14½ oz) fat-free chicken broth
1	can (15 oz) chickpeas, drained
¼	tsp hot-pepper sauce
¼	c chopped parsley

1. Cook the sausage in a deep nonstick skillet over medium-high heat until no longer pink inside, about 6 minutes. Drain on paper towels to remove the excess fat. Place in a colander, and pour boiling water over it. Drain well.

2. Heat the oil in the same skillet over medium heat. Add the onions, and cook until soft, about 10 minutes. Stir in the peppers, garlic, oregano, herbes de Provence, and paprika. Cook for 7 minutes. Stir in the tomatoes (with juice), broth, chickpeas, hot pepper sauce, and sausage. Simmer for 8 minutes. Stir in the parsley, and serve.

Makes 6 servings

Per serving: 259 cal, 12 g pro, 22 g carb, 14 g fat, 4 g sat. fat, 29 mg chol, 5 g fiber, 1,042 mg sodium

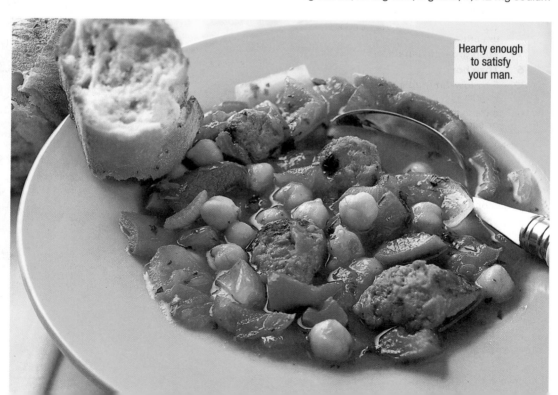

Hearty enough to satisfy your man.

Shrimp with Greens and Red Beans

Prepare your plate (and your palate) for a seafood dish that's full of flavor—and onions, peppers, Swiss chard, and kidney beans too. Health bonus: Each serving provides plenty of fiber and a bit of omega-3 fats—both of which are good for protecting your heart.

4	cloves garlic, minced
1½	tsp ground paprika
1	tsp dried thyme, crushed
½	tsp ground black pepper
¼	tsp salt
¼	tsp ground red pepper
1	lb lg shrimp, peeled and deveined
2	Tbsp olive oil
2	ribs celery, thinly sliced
1	lg onion, chopped
1	lg green bell pepper, chopped
¾	c chicken broth
3	c green or red Swiss chard, thinly sliced
1	can (14–19 oz) red kidney beans

1. In a medium bowl, combine the garlic and spices. Remove about half of the mixture to a small bowl. Add the shrimp to the medium bowl, and toss to coat well.

2. Heat the oil in a large saucepan or Dutch oven over medium heat. Add the celery, onion, and green pepper. Cook, stirring frequently, for 6 minutes, or until crisp-tender.

3. Add the reserved spice mixture, and cook, stirring frequently, for 2 minutes. Add ¼ cup of the broth. Cover, and cook, stirring often, for 5 minutes.

4. Add the chard, and cook, stirring frequently, for 2 minutes, or until wilted. Stir in the beans, shrimp, and the remaining ½ cup broth, and bring to a boil over high heat. Reduce the heat to low, cover, and simmer for 4 minutes, or until the shrimp are opaque.

Makes 4 servings
Per serving: 306 cal, 31 g pro, 26 g carb, 9 g fat, 1 g sat. fat, 172 mg chol, 9 g fiber, 733 mg sodium

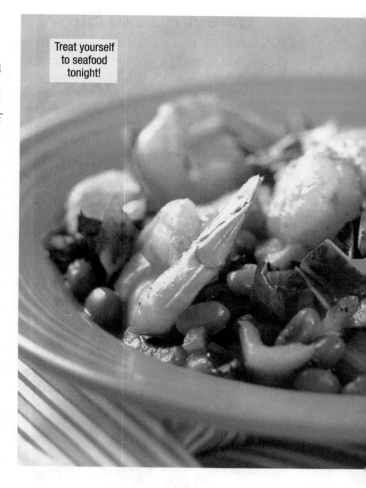

Treat yourself to seafood tonight!

‖ Sweet Potato Stew

Ladle yourself a bowl of this unique stew! It's packed with some of the sweetest veggies, including sweet potatoes and red bell peppers. Health bonus: This meal is rich in iron and vitamin C, two nutrients that help your body fight stress and fatigue.

1½	c brown rice
1	Tbsp olive oil
3	cloves garlic, minced
2	red bell peppers, cut into 1" chunks
1	lg onion, chopped
1	Tbsp chopped fresh ginger
½	tsp ground allspice
¼	tsp ground red pepper
4	c vegetable broth
2	lg sweet potatoes, peeled and cut into 1" chunks
½	c natural peanut butter
1	c boiling water
⅓	c tomato paste
1	can (10½–15 oz) chickpeas, rinsed and drained
1	lb spinach, coarsely chopped

1. Prepare the rice per package directions.

2. Meanwhile, heat the oil in a Dutch oven over medium-high heat. Add the garlic, bell peppers, and onion. Cook for 3 minutes. Add the ginger, allspice, and ground red pepper. Cook for 1 minute.

3. Add the broth and sweet potatoes, and bring to a boil. Reduce the heat to low, cover, and simmer for 15 minutes.

4. In a bowl, whisk the peanut butter and water. Add to the Dutch oven along with the tomato paste, chickpeas, and spinach. Cook for 10 minutes, or until heated through. Serve over the rice.

Makes 6 servings

Per serving: 426 cal, 19 g pro, 61 g carb, 16 g fat, 3 g sat. fat, 0 mg chol, 16 g fiber, 669 mg sodium

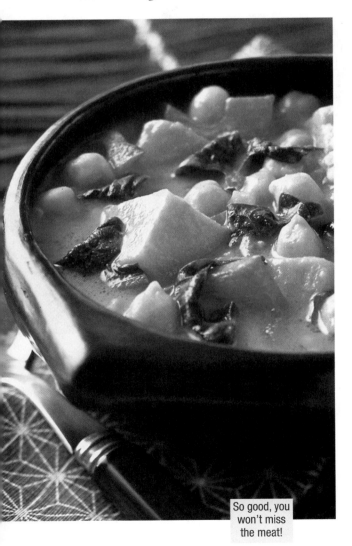

So good, you won't miss the meat!

Penne with Zucchini-Garlic Sauce

Here we topped one of your favorite pastas with flavorful zucchini to give you an extra helping of vegetables in a delicious, gourmet-style sauce. Health bonus: Zucchini is one of the lowest-calorie foods in existence. It also contributes a good amount of fiber, along with some potassium, magnesium, and a little vitamin C and folate.

4	med zucchini, about 1½ lb
4	Tbsp garlic olive oil*
8	oz penne pasta

1. Wash the zucchini, and cut 1½ of them into thick rounds. Cut the rounds in half, and place them in a small saucepan. Add enough salted water to just cover. Bring to a boil. Lower the heat, and cover the pan. Cook for 15 minutes.

2. Using a slotted spoon, transfer the zucchini to a blender. Add ½ cup of the cooking water and 1 teaspoon of the oil. Process until very smooth. Add salt and ground black pepper to taste. Set aside.

3. Trim off the ends of the remaining zucchini, and discard. Cut the zucchini into ¼" cubes.

4. Heat the remaining oil in a large nonstick skillet, add the zucchini cubes, and sauté over high heat until the zucchini softens and turns golden, about 8 minutes. Add salt and pepper to taste.

5. Bring a large pot of salted water to a boil. Add the pasta, and cook until tender.

6. Drain the pasta thoroughly. Divide among 4 shallow soup bowls. Distribute the cooked zucchini and oil evenly over the pasta. Heat the zucchini-garlic sauce, and pour over the pasta. Add a little pepper. Serve immediately.

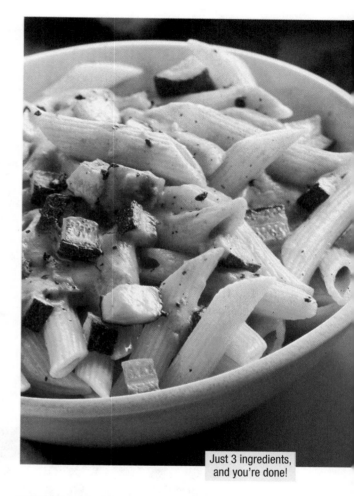

Just 3 ingredients, and you're done!

Makes 4 servings
Per serving: (with ½ teaspoon added salt) 354 cal, 9 g pro, 47 g carb, 15 g fat, 2 g sat. fat, 0 mg chol, 4 g fiber, 240 mg sodium

*To make garlic olive oil, place 1 cup olive oil in a small saucepan. Add 8 cloves garlic, and cook over medium heat until small bubbles form on the surface. Cook 5 minutes longer. Remove from the heat, and let it sit for 2 hours. Strain into a clean jar. Cover, and refrigerate.

Roasted Eggplant Italian

If you like fried eggplant Parmesan, you'll love this baked variation. It's high in Italian flavor and low in fat and calories! Health bonus: This veggie-rich dish is a great source of vitamins A and C and calcium.

2	**Tbsp canola oil**
1	**eggplant (1½ lb), peeled and sliced lengthwise 1/4" thick**
½	**c chopped onion**
1	**can (16 oz) diced tomatoes**
1	**c reduced-fat or fat-free ricotta**
1	**c coarsely chopped spinach**
¼	**c reduced-fat mozzarella**
1	**Tbsp dried basil**
1	**Tbsp dried oregano**
1	**tsp garlic powder**
1	**c tomato sauce**

1. Preheat the oven to 350°F. Brush 1 tablespoon of the oil on the sliced eggplant, and roast it until tender, about 15 minutes.

2. Sauté the onion in the remaining 1 tablespoon of the oil until tender, about 3 to 4 minutes. Add the tomatoes (with juice), and simmer for 15 minutes.

3. In a separate bowl, mix the ricotta, spinach, mozzarella, basil, oregano, and garlic. Add salt and pepper to taste.

4. Lightly coat a baking dish with cooking spray. Spoon the cheese mixture on each slice of the eggplant, and roll up like a jelly roll. Place the eggplant rolls in the baking dish. Continue until all the eggplant is used.

5. Top with the tomato sauce, and bake for 30 minutes.

Makes 4 servings
Per serving: 251 cal, 13 g pro, 23 g carb, 13 g fat, 4 g sat. fat, 23 mg chol, 6 g fiber, 330 mg sodium

Editor's note: Not long ago, eggplants were bitter and had to be salted to draw out their bitter juices before cooking. Thanks to new farming methods, eggplants no longer contain these bitter juices, so you can skip this step when cooking with them.

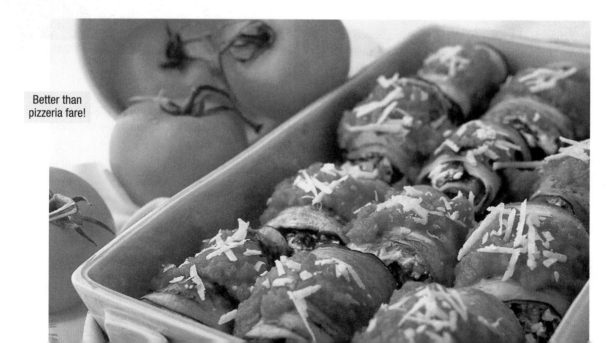

Better than pizzeria fare!

Spaghetti Squash Marinara

Pasta lovers will crave this wonderful all-vegetable dish made with spaghetti squash, which is lower in calories than regular pasta. Health bonus: You'll get a good amount of fiber and cancer-fighting lycopene in each serving.

1	med spaghetti squash
2	Tbsp olive oil
1	lg Spanish (yellow) onion, cut into long, thin strips
1	clove garlic, finely chopped
1	sm zucchini, cut into ¼-4" strips
1	sm yellow squash, cut into ¼-4" strips
1	med red bell pepper, seeded, and cut into ¼-4" strips
2	c canned tomato puree
1	c loosely packed fresh basil leaves
½	tsp salt
⅛	tsp ground black pepper

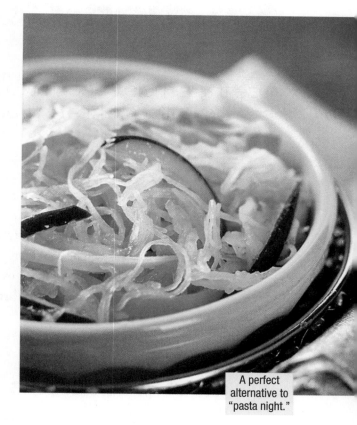

A perfect alternative to "pasta night."

1. Prick the spaghetti squash all over with a fork. Place it in a microwaveable dish, and microwave on high for 15 to 20 minutes, or until it softens. Remove from the microwave, and let it cool. (Be careful; it gets very hot.)

2. When the squash is cool enough to handle, halve it lengthwise. Then scrape out the seeds, and throw them away. Set the squash aside.

3. Warm 1 tablespoon of the oil in a 4- to 6-quart pot over medium heat. Add the onion and garlic, and cook, stirring often, for about 10 minutes, or until the onion starts to brown. Add water, 1 tablespoon at a time, as necessary to prevent burning. Add the remaining 1 tablespoon oil, zucchini, yellow squash, and bell pepper to the pot, and cook for about 10 minutes, or until the vegetables soften slightly.

4. Add the tomato puree and basil, and simmer over low heat for about 15 minutes.

5. While the sauce is simmering, gently remove the spaghetti squash strands using 2 forks, and add them to the sauce. Stir in the salt and pepper, and cook for 1 to 2 minutes longer, or until the squash is heated through.

Makes 8 servings

Per serving: 97 cal, 3 g pro, 16 g carb, 4 g fat, 1 g sat. fat, 0 mg chol, 4 g fiber, 386 mg sodium

Your 4-Week Portion-Control Planner

Use this simple checklist to help you keep your new healthy eating habits on track

Slipping into a healthy lifestyle just got easier than ever, and soon slipping into a smaller pair of jeans will be too! Here, you'll find an easy-to-use planner to help guide you, motivate you, and cheer you on over the next 4 weeks. Our goal? To help you put to use the simple eating advice from Part One. So grab a pen, and get ready to "X" your way to a smaller size starting *today*!

Quick Reminder about Food Portions

Here's a simple review of how to divide up your plate at breakfast, lunch, and dinner. For more details on this plan for weight loss, see Chapter 2. You'll also find some great meal ideas there, as well as in Chapter 6. Remember: At lunchtime, use an 8" plate. Save the 10" plates for dinnertime.

At every meal:
- ▶ ½ plate = fruits and vegetables
- ▶ ¼ plate = protein (fish, beans, low-fat dairy, or lean meats)
- ▶ ¼ plate = starch (whole grains or beans)

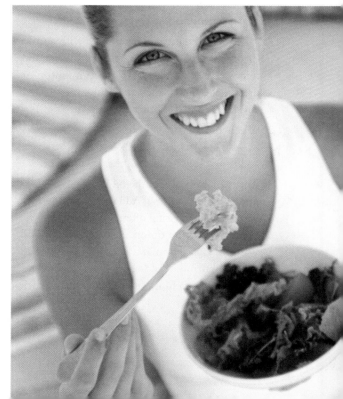

Remember: Half that plate should be veggies!

44

Your Daily Food Checklist

Put an "X" in the appropriate box every time you follow healthy portion-control habits.

WEEK ONE

	Monday	Tuesday	Wednesday	Thursday	Friday	Saturday	Sunday
Breakfast							
Lunch							
Dinner							
Snacks							

WEEK TWO

	Monday	Tuesday	Wednesday	Thursday	Friday	Saturday	Sunday
Breakfast							
Lunch							
Dinner							
Snacks							

WEEK THREE

	Monday	Tuesday	Wednesday	Thursday	Friday	Saturday	Sunday
Breakfast							
Lunch							
Dinner							
Snacks							

WEEK FOUR

	Monday	Tuesday	Wednesday	Thursday	Friday	Saturday	Sunday
Breakfast							
Lunch							
Dinner							
Snacks							

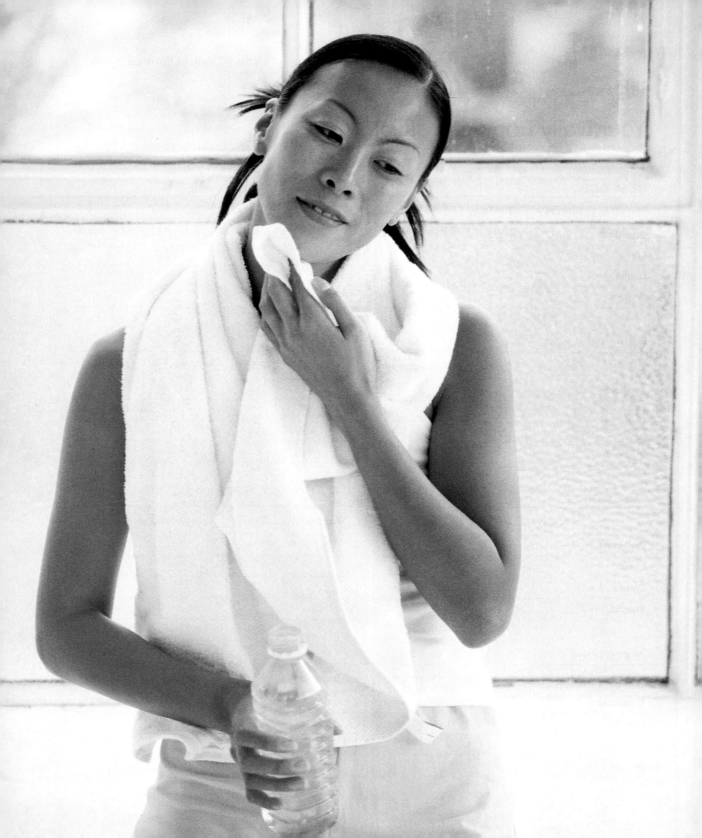

PART TWO

Quickie Workouts— Fast Results!

CHAPTER 7

Fit and Firm in 8 Minutes a Day!

This easy at-home strength training workout will get you fit in next to no time!

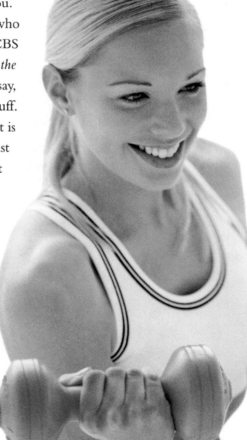

If you don't want to spend hours in the gym but want to look as if you do, this program is for you.

Jorge Cruise is a certified personal trainer who has been featured on *Oprah*, Lifetime TV, CBS news, and ABC news. His book, *8 Minutes in the Morning*, is a national bestseller. Suffice it to say, when it comes to working out, he knows his stuff.

If you want a strength training workout that is both effective *and* quick, you'll be amazed at just how little time you'll have to put in—and just how fast you'll get results. Cruise's program is the result of his coaching more than 3 million people online. He created it based on their feedback and success stories specifically for people who are time-deprived but

Weights do things aerobics class can't!

want rapid results. "When I suggest to people that they get up 8 minutes earlier in the morning to exercise, I sometimes get, 'Oh, I'm not a morning person,'" says Cruise. "But I truly believe that's all in your head. I used to stay up late at night because I thought of myself as a night owl. So when I first started exercising in the morning, I had a really tough time doing it consistently." But, asserts Cruise, there are two great reasons to change your sleeping habits.

It will help you stick with it. Morning is the only time of day that most people have free. Later, distractions will come up. You may plan to do your exercises during a lunch break, but a friend asks you to lunch, and you think, "Okay, I'll do them after work." But, after work, your 10-year-old asks for help with his homework. Then your husband wants to snuggle on the couch. According to research, morning exercisers have a better stick-with-it rate. When you commit to exercising in the morning, you bypass excuses.

That feels good. Exercising sends a signal to your pituitary gland to release endorphins, your body's natural feel-good drug. The more endorphins you have in your bloodstream, the better you feel. When you exercise in the morning, you will feel better and handle yourself better no matter what happens in your day, whether it's getting stuck in a traffic jam, dealing with a cranky coworker, or tending to a sick child.

No, Aerobics Aren't Enough!

Although aerobic exercise is essential for strengthening your heart and lungs, by itself, it is not the

I Replaced Channel Surfing with Weight Lifting—and Lost 45 Lb!

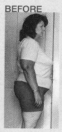 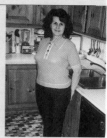

BEFORE

"I figured that I would try his program because 8 minutes was less time than I spent flipping through channels during TV commercials. Day by day, I got fitter, and I lost weight," says Ann-Marie Carpenter, who lost 45 lb, thanks to these strength-training moves.

most effective way to get lean. If you focus only on aerobics, your overall body shape will stay the same, even if you burn fat. For example, if you are pear-shaped, and you do only aerobic exercise, you will just look like a smaller pear. And your body will still be flabby.

By doing the exercises in the "8 Minutes in the Morning" workout, you will both burn fat and improve your body shape. You will tone your shoulders so that your waist looks narrower. Your arms will be smaller as well as firmer. Your abdominal muscles will not only be leaner but also stronger, and as a result, they'll provide better support for your torso.

That's not to say you shouldn't do any aerobics. *Prevention* magazine recommends that you do about 30 minutes of aerobics every day to keep your heart and lungs strong. Plus, it helps to reduce your stress level. See Chapter 8 for a simple walking workout that can do all that and more.

More Benefits of Strength Training

Working with weights does far more than firm your body. Here are a few more perks to "sell" you on the idea of strength training.

You'll burn more calories. An important factor that determines how much fat you burn throughout the day is the amount of lean muscle tissue in your body. The more lean muscle tissue you have, the more efficiently your body burns fat. Lean tissue derives 75 to 95% of its energy from body fat, so for every new pound of muscle you build, you incinerate about 30 additional calories per day. The more lean tissue you have, the more body fat you will shed—even at night, while you sleep. For example, if two women weigh the same amount but one has 5 lb more muscle, she will burn an extra 150 calories a day.

You'll lose more fat. Normally when you lose weight, you lose 75% of it as fat and 25% of it as muscle. But when you do strength training, you lose nearly *all* fat and no muscle.

You'll look and feel younger. Strength training turns back the aging clock. Not only does it make you stronger so that everything you do is easier, but it also builds bone, helps you shed fat, and increases your muscle mass, so you'll feel healthier.

You'll be more active all day long. Once your muscles become stronger—usually by week 2 or 3—you will find yourself suddenly doing things you never thought possible. You'll take a walk instead of sitting in front of the TV, take the stairs instead of the elevator, and take quick walking breaks instead of sitting at your desk all day. All of this will accelerate your results.

The "8 Minutes in the Morning" Workout

Start with a short warm-up. Do one set of 12 repetitions from exercise A, then immediately do one set of 12 reps from exercise B. Switch back to exercise A, and continue the cycle for a total of four sets. If you can do an exercise more than 12 times, the weight is too light. If you can't reach 12 repetitions, the weight is too heavy. Cool down, and stretch when you're finished.

Equipment Checklist

Before you can put this program into action, you'll need to have a few "gym" items at home. In addition to needing an exercise mat to cushion your body for the floor exercises in this chapter, you'll need a chair (for Day 1 and Day 4) and some dumbbells of varying weights. If you don't already have dumbbells, take this book along to the sporting goods store, and use some 5-lb dumbbells to try each of the exercises in this chapter. If you can do more than 12 repetitions with that weight, move up to a slightly heavier weight. When you find one that you can *only* do 12 reps with, that's the one you want. You may need to purchase several different weights of dumbbells if some of your muscle groups are stronger than others. Remember: The money you spend on equipment will help offset future medical costs by keeping you healthier.

Day 1

EXERCISE A
CHEST

Dumbbell Press: Lie on a mat on your back with your knees bent and your feet flat on the floor. You may place one or more pillows under your back and head for support. Holding a dumbbell in each hand, bring your elbows in line with your shoulders, making a right angle between your upper arm and your side. Exhale as you slowly extend your arms and press the dumbbells toward the ceiling. Keep your elbows loose. Hold for 1 second. Inhale as you return to the starting point.

EXERCISE B
BACK

Two-Arm Row: Sit in a chair, and grasp a dumbbell in each hand. You may put a pillow on your lap for support. Lean forward, and extend your arms straight down, being sure to keep your elbows loose. Exhale as you slowly bring your elbows toward the ceiling. Once the dumbbells reach the top of your thighs, hold for 1 second. Inhale as you slowly lower the dumbbells.

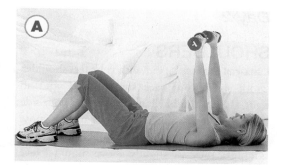

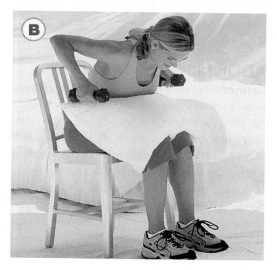

IT WORKED FOR ME!

I Traded Fatigue for Fitness— and Lost 15 Lb!

"When I first started this program, I felt unfit and fatigued. But each week, I lost an average of 2 lb. I was soon standing straighter and had more bounce in my walk. Now I feel terrific, and my morning workouts start my day off on the right track," says Jill Leonard, who lost 15 lb.

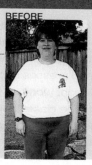

BEFORE

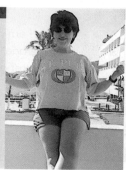

Day 2

EXERCISE A
SHOULDERS

Lateral Raise: Stand with your feet shoulder-width apart, your back straight, and your abs tight. Hold a dumbbell in each hand at your sides with your arms straight and your elbows loose. Exhale as you slowly lift the dumbbells out to the side until they are slightly above shoulder level and your palms are facing the floor. Hold for 1 second. Inhale as you lower your arms.

EXERCISE B
ABDOMINALS

Crunch: Lie on a mat on your back with your knees bent and your feet flat on the floor. Make a fist with your right hand, and place it between your chin and collarbone. With your left hand, grasp your right wrist. This will prevent you from leading with your head and straining your neck. Without moving your lower body, exhale, and slowly curl your upper torso until your shoulder blades are off the floor. Hold for 1 second. Inhale as you slowly lower yourself.

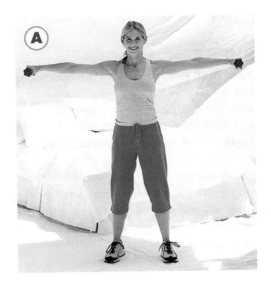

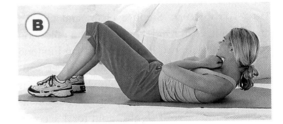

IT WORKED FOR ME!

I Lift Weights with a Group—and Firmed My Whole Body!

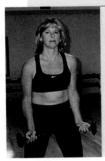

"I am not the self-motivated type," says Shawni Littlehale, 42. So instead of "going it alone" with a weight workout, Shawni joined a group strength training class. In this type of strength training, an instructor leads a group of people through exercises such as curls, rows, and presses using dumbbells, bars, or resistance bands. Compared with a traditional weight workout, the emphasis is on lighter weights (3 to 8 lb) and more repetitions.

"With the class, there's kind of a camaraderie," says Shawni. "You feel like you're in it together, obligated to get there every week and chart mutual progress."

Day 3

EXERCISE A
TRICEPS (BACK OF ARMS)

Lying Kickback: Lie on a mat on your back with a dumbbell in each hand by your ears and the dumbbells pointing toward the ceiling. Straighten your arms, but keep your elbows loose. Hold for 1 second. Inhale as you return to the starting point.

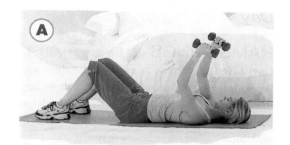

EXERCISE B
BICEPS (FRONT OF ARMS)

Standing Curl: Stand with your feet shoulder-width apart. Hold a dumbbell in each hand at your sides with your arms extended. Exhale as you simultaneously curl both arms to just past 90 degrees, bringing your palms toward your biceps. Keep your elbows close to your sides, and concentrate on moving only from your elbow joints, not from your shoulders. Hold arms in the "curled" position for 1 second. Inhale as you lower.

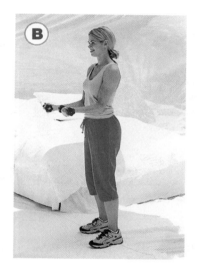

Instead of resting between exercises, you're moving constantly, with calisthenics and stretches mixed in. The upbeat music helps keep you going, so your heart rate stays up. It also burns 204 to 408 calories an hour (based on a 150-lb person).

Since trying group strength training, Shawni has noticed that she is leaner, her waist is slimmer, and her clothes fit better. She also lost about 5 lb in the first 4 months, but since muscle weighs more than fat, she has probably trimmed down even more than the scale reflects.

Getting started: To find a group strength training class, call local health clubs and gyms. This type of weight workout is perfect for beginners: It's a good way to get started without feeling intimidated, and the instructor can make sure that you're performing each exercise correctly.

Day 4

EXERCISE A
HAMSTRINGS (BACK OF THIGHS)

Leg Lift: Lie with your back on the floor and your heels on the seat of a chair. Exhale as you slowly contract the back of your upper thighs to push your butt toward the ceiling. Hold for 1 second. Inhale as you slowly lower your butt.

EXERCISE B
QUADRICEPS (FRONT OF THIGHS)

Squat: Stand with your feet slightly wider than shoulder-width apart. Keeping your back straight and your abs tight, exhale as you slowly squat down to about 90°. Don't let your knees extend past your toes. Make sure to push your butt out as if you were sitting in a chair. Hold for 1 second. Inhale as you slowly return to the starting position.

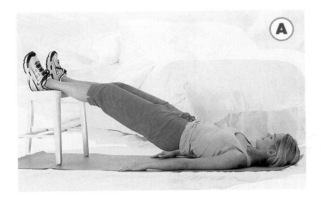

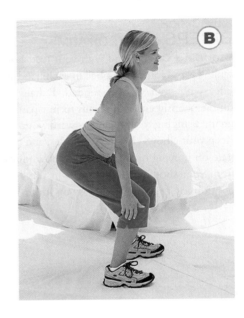

Fit and firm muscles will help you be more active and energetic all the time.

DO JUST ONE THING!
Have Backup Plans

If, by some fluke, you miss your morning workout, *immediately* plan your workout for later during the day—but also be sure you have a Plan B and C, especially if your schedule is routinely disrupted. For instance, you may want to carry exercise bands or keep a set of dumbbells in your trunk for lunchtime workouts. Then, if you wind up working through lunch, plan to do your resistance training before commuting home. You may even miss some of the rush hour traffic!

Day 5

EXERCISE A
CALVES

Standing Raise: Stand with your feet shoulder-width apart. Hold a dumbbell in each hand, allowing them to hang comfortably at your sides and keeping your arms extended but not locked. Keep your chest out, your shoulder blades rolled back and down, and your abdominal muscles tight. Exhale as you slowly lift your heels and rise onto your toes. Hold for 1 second. Inhale as you slowly lower.

EXERCISE B
BUTT

Kick-Up: Kneel on all fours with your knees hip-width apart, your hands slightly wider apart than your shoulders, and your fingers pointing forward. Keep your back straight and your head up. Raise your right leg until your thigh is in line with your torso. Exhale as you slowly push your foot toward the ceiling. Once you've reached your maximum contraction, hold for 1 second. Inhale as you slowly lower your leg until it is once again in line with your torso. Do 12 lifts using your right leg, then do 12 lifts using your left leg. That equals one set.

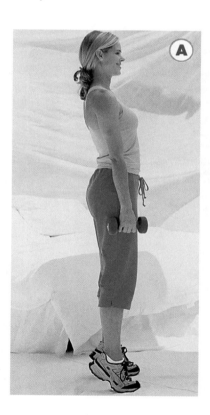

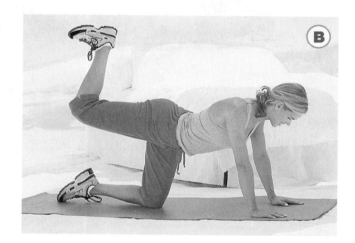

When you do strength training,
you lose nearly *all* fat and no muscle.

Day 6

EXERCISE A
INNER THIGH

Inner-Thigh Leg Raise: Lie on your left side with your left elbow and forearm supporting your upper body and your left leg extended. Bend your right knee, and place your right foot behind your left leg for balance. Keeping your left leg straight, exhale as you slowly lift your left foot as high as you can. Hold for 1 second. Inhale as you lower your foot back to the starting position. Do one set with your left leg, then switch sides.

EXERCISE B
OUTER THIGH

Doggie: Kneel on all fours with your knees hip-width apart, your hands slightly wider apart than your shoulders, and your fingers pointing forward. Keep your back straight and your head up. Keeping your leg bent at a 90° angle, exhale as you raise your right leg out to the side. Hold for 1 second. Inhale as you slowly lower your leg back to the starting point. Do one set with your right leg, then switch sides.

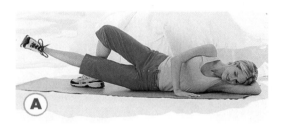

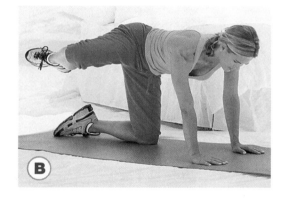

Exercise in the AM, and you won't ever have to miss a workout.

CHAPTER 8

Your Turn-Up-the-Burn Walking Workout

Three great programs that burn calories, beat boredom, and kick calorie burning into high gear!

It's no secret that walking is great for shedding pounds. Not only does it burn calories and tone up your muscles, it's also gentle and low-impact, which makes it easier on the body than many other aerobic activities. And studies show that while running and swimming may burn more calories than walking, people who take up walking tend to be better about sticking with the program for weeks, months, and even years.

Beyond being a great weight loss tool, walking also gets your heart pumping to help improve cardiovascular fitness, and it helps keep your bones strong as the years go by. Walking doesn't require any gear besides a pair of good walking shoes, and you can do it just about anywhere—on a treadmill, in your neighborhood, in a park, or even in the mall! What's

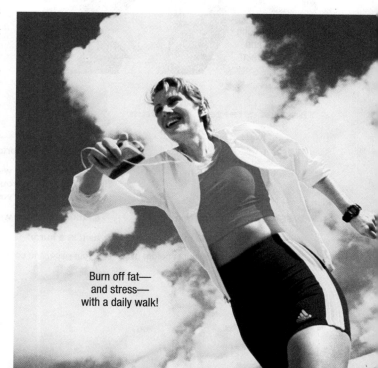

Burn off fat—
and stress—
with a daily walk!

more, it's a great way to lower your stress level—especially if you use the time to focus on the beauty of nature instead of rehashing the day's events. Once you've been walking regularly for a few weeks, chances are you'll even find a few walking benefits we've missed!

If you're new to walking, you'll want to try the Get-Started Program that follows: After 4 weeks, you should notice the pounds melting away! Once that workout becomes too easy—or if you've already been walking for a while and have hit a weight loss plateau—move on to The Turn-Up-the-Burn Program on p. 60 to start the numbers on the scale moving downward again! Last, we've included a run/walk program on p. 62 to help boost your metabolism a little bit more and ease you into running, if that's your goal. Choose the program that's right for you—then get out there and do it!

The Get-Started Program

Choose this program if any one of the following statements rings true for you:

- ▶ You're severely overweight.
- ▶ You're recovering from illness or surgery.
- ▶ You have a chronic health problem that limits activity.
- ▶ You devote less than 60 minutes a day to "active" tasks such as walking the dog, chasing after kids, or putting out the garbage.
- ▶ You spend your days sitting at a desk or in your car and your evenings sitting on the couch.

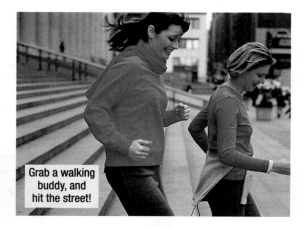
Grab a walking buddy, and hit the street!

The Get-Started Program

	Duration	Speed	Frequency
WEEK 1	10 min.	whatever is comfortable	3 days/week
WEEK 2	15 min.	a little faster than week 1; after walking 10 min., you should have gone farther than you did last week	4 days/week
WEEK 3	20 min.	a little faster than week 2	5 days/week
WEEK 4	30 min.	as if in a hurry*	5 days/week

*Be sure to stroll for 5 minutes before picking up your pace, and cool down with a 5-minute stroll at the end of your workout.

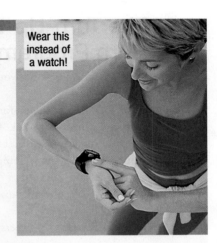

Wear this instead of a watch!

DO JUST ONE THING!
Check Your Heart Rate

You can exercise longer and burn more fat if you're in your target heart rate zone—not too easy, not too hard. "One reason people quit exercising is that they push themselves too hard and feel fatigued or get injured," says Ed Burke, PhD, author of *Precision Heart Rate Training* (Human Kinetics, 1998). Likewise, some fail to see results because they never work hard enough. Tracking how many beats per minute (BPM) your heart pumps during exercise helps you adjust your workouts to maximize benefits.

To get your target heart rate zone, subtract your age from 220. That's your maximum heart rate (MHR). For best results, exercise within 60 to 80% of your MHR. If you're age 40, your MHR is 180 BPM (220 − 40), and your target range is 108 to 144 BPM (180 × .60; 180 × .80). Remember: This is just a rough estimate. Always consider how you feel too.

To check your heart rate, take your pulse at your wrist or neck. Or for an easier, more accurate reading, try a heart rate monitor, available at sporting goods stores.

With the Get-Started Program, you'll gradually build up to a regular walking routine. This program starts you out slowly, which will help build your confidence and reduce your risk of injury. You'll reap plenty of benefits even at a moderate pace (in which you're moving fast enough to get your heart pumping, but you're not out of breath). Almost immediately, you'll notice improvements in your flexibility, your energy level, and your mood. After the second week of the program, your workouts will feel easier—a sign that your heart is getting fitter, and your legs are getting stronger.

Sticking to It

Once you start walking, the next challenge is to stick with it. Here are some tips to keep you on track.

Count all the benefits. Losing weight is a great motivator, but don't overlook the other benefits, among them: stress reduction, improved mood, better-fitting clothes, leftover energy in the evening, and more.

Take it all in. While you're walking, breathe in the fresh air, smell fragrant plants, and watch birds and animals.

Start surfing the 'net. A little encouragement goes a long way. Walking with friends is a sure way to keep you moving. But if that's not possible, try the next best thing: virtual walking buddies. To join a walking discussion group, surf your way to www.walkingfit.com.

The Turn-Up-the-Burn Program

This workout is ideal for you if you can relate to some of the following:

▶ Your scale hasn't budged for a month.

▶ You've been doing week 4 of the Get-Started Program for at least 6 weeks.

▶ You're bored with walking, and you're starting to skip workouts.

▶ You don't have a formal exercise routine, but your days are active.

When you first started fitness walking, the going was tougher, and the pounds came off relatively quickly. Now that you've built up your strength and stamina, you'll need to boost the intensity of your workout to *keep* losing weight. The problem is, walking at a quicker pace for your entire workout could lead to injuries. That's why this walking program has you increase your workout's intensity by adding short bursts of quicker walking throughout your workout.

Sticking to It

It's really hard to stick with any exercise program when you're not seeing immediate results. Here's

---

IT WORKED FOR ME!

"I Climbed a Mountain—and Reached New Fitness Heights!"

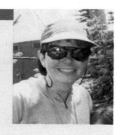

"Before I turned 40, I was stressed and out of shape," says Linda Millman Josephson, a mother of three. Then she took up mountain climbing. "I was intrigued by the simplicity. I was under a ton of stress, but committing to one goal put things in perspective."

At first, Linda was worried about being able to make it up a mountain, in part because of her bad knees, so she had a trainer help her build leg strength. After 10 months of weight training and stair stepping twice a week, weekend hikes, and training climbs, Linda was prepared to head for the summit of Mt. Rainier (14,410 ft).

"We started out at 11 AM, arriving in late afternoon at our camp, where we tried to get a few hours of rest. Then, in the dead of the night, we started our final ascent. The mountain was eerie and unbelievably beautiful, quiet, and glowing blue. It was like being on another planet!" says Linda. At dawn, she finally reached the summit.

That wasn't her only accomplishment, though. In the process of training, she dropped four dress sizes too!

"I've gone from thinking that my body isn't capable to finding out that it is," she asserts. "Now I'm much more willing to try new things."

Getting started: If you're interested in taking your workout to new heights, talk to staffers at your local recreation departments and outdoor recreation or sporting goods stores. They are good resources for group hikes, trails, and instruction in climbing.

The Turn-Up-the-Burn Program

	Duration	Speed	Frequency
WEEK 1	5 min.	stroll (warm-up)	5 days/week
	5 min.	normal walk	
	5 min.	as if in a hurry	
	10 min.	normal walk (recover)	
	5 min.	as if in a hurry	
	5 min.	stroll (cool-down)	
WEEK 2	5 min.	stroll (warm-up)	5 days/week
	5 min.	normal walk	
	5 min.	as if in a hurry; after walking 10 min., you should have gone farther than you did last week	
	10 min.	normal walk (recover)	
	5 min.	as if in a hurry (again moving faster than in week 1)	
	5 min.	stroll (cool-down)	
WEEK 3	5 min.	stroll (warm-up)	5 days/week
	5 min.	normal walk	
	5 min.	as if in a hurry (same pace as week 2)	
	8 min.	normal walk (recover)	
	5 min.	as if in a hurry	
	7 min.	normal walk (recover)	
	5 min.	as if in a hurry	
	5 min.	stroll (cool-down)	
WEEK 4	5 min.	stroll (warm-up)	5 days/week
	5 min.	as if in a hurry (same pace as week 3)	
	5 min.	normal walk (recover)	
	5 min.	as if in a hurry	
	5 min.	normal walk (recover)	
	5 min.	as if in a hurry	
	5 min.	normal walk (recover)	
	5 min.	as if in a hurry	
	5 min.	stroll (cool-down)	

how to stay motivated until the pounds start to come off again.

Indulge yourself! Walks are your very own time. Relax, take deep breaths, dream—and when stressful thoughts start to creep in, redirect your mind back toward happy topics.

Vary your route. Walk somewhere beautiful, such as a hiking trail, along a river, or in a park. Or plan a walking vacation to places such as the lush, green New England countryside or the sunny California coast. The anticipation will keep you walking.

Keep a mileage log. As you pick up speed, you'll be able to go farther. Keep a log of how many miles (or how many minutes) you walk, then reward yourself when you top the pre- vious week's "record." You can use the chart on p. 79 to keep track of your achievements, or check your local bookstore for a log book designed specifically for runners or walkers.

The Run-Walk Program

This workout is just what you need if you agree with any of these statements:

▶ You think walking is too easy.
▶ You want to lose weight fast.
▶ You've been walking for 30 minutes, 5 days a week, for at least 6 weeks.
▶ You want to trade walking for running.

The Right Shoes for Run-Walking

Before you add bouts of running to your daily walks, take a look at what you put on your feet. When you run, your feet are briefly airborne. When they hit the ground again, the impact on your body is two to three times harder than when you're just walking. This puts you at

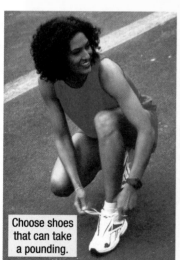

Choose shoes that can take a pounding.

greater risk for injury, says Howard Palamarchuk, DPM, of Temple University School of Podiatric Medicine in Philadelphia. So what should you wear to run-walk? "You can't go wrong with a running shoe," he says. You really need the extra cushion that a running shoe provides, more than any special feature that you'll find in a walking shoe.

What to look for in a running shoe: Higher heel elevation and a dual-density midsole to control the extra foot motion (look for two colors at the heel) are best. Also important is flexibility in the forefoot (look for grooves on the bottom of the shoe near the ball of the foot, or try bending the ends together to make sure the shoe bends at the front, not the middle).

You can also try a run/walk hybrid shoe, found in specialty stores. Footwear companies are beginning to cater to the run-walk market.

The Run-Walk Program

	Speed/Duration *	Repetitions	Frequency
WEEK 1	Run 2 min.; walk 4 min.	Repeat 5×	4 days/week
WEEK 2	Run 3 min.; walk 3 min.	Repeat 5×	4 days/week
WEEK 3	Run 5 min.; walk 2.5 min.	Repeat 4×	4 days/week
WEEK 4	Run 7 min.; walk 3 min.	Repeat 3×	4 days/week
WEEK 5	Run 8 min.; walk 2 min.	Repeat 3×	4 days/week
WEEK 6	Run 9 min.; walk 2 min.	Repeat 2×, then run 8 min.	4 days/week
WEEK 7	Run 9 min.; walk 1 min.	Repeat 3×	4 days/week
WEEK 8	Run 13 min.; walk 2 min.	Repeat 2×	4 days/week
WEEK 9	Run 14 min.; walk 1 min.	Repeat 2×	4 days/week
WEEK 10	Run 30 min.	—	4 days/week

*Be sure to warm up for 5 minutes before beginning your run-walk routine, and cool down for 5 minutes at the end of your workout.

Want to burn more calories and fat while you walk? Add a bit of running to the mix! Even just a few minutes of running during your walks can help you burn more calories, build stronger bones, and boost your fitness level. With this versatile program, you can do the full 10 weeks, which will leave you running for 30 minutes at a time. Or if you just want to add a little speedwork to your program, stop at whatever level feels comfortable to you. Note: If you feel tired after completing week 7, repeat the week 7 program again before moving on to week 8. Also be sure to take a day of rest between the first three sessions to give your body time to recover.

Sticking To It

Here are a few ways to keep your run-walk workouts on schedule.

Let music guide your intervals. Instead of constantly checking your watch to figure out when to run and when to walk, record upbeat music, and then add a voice cue on the tape to mark when you should change pace.

Choose a fitting reward. Buy a new workout outfit, or treat yourself to a massage for not missing a workout in a whole week.

Sign up and train for a race. You'll be motivated to stick with the program—especially if you take pledges, and people are counting on you to finish!

CHAPTER 9

Our Best Belly-Flattening Plan Ever!

This breakthrough program uses new science to help you get great results—guaranteed!

Most women do ab exercises for one reason alone: to flatten their tummy. But did you know that these moves can do much more than give you a bikini-worthy belly? Strong abdominal muscles also

▶ protect your back from injury and pain

▶ help you maintain proper posture (which slims your silhouette even more)

▶ let you effortlessly perform activities that require bending and twisting, such as hoisting grocery bags out of your car

"Your trunk muscles form the core through which all forces are transferred, whether that's absorbing the ground's impact while walking, gathering power to throw a ball or swing a racket, or resisting gravity, so you can stand tall," says

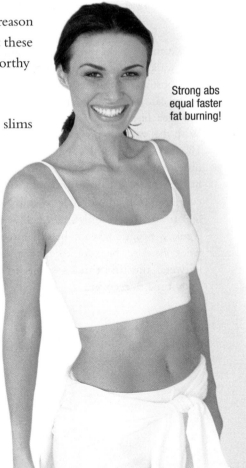

Strong abs equal faster fat burning!

Prevention fitness advisor Wayne L. Westcott, PhD. Stronger core muscles also rev up your metabolism, so you lose fat faster. That's important, because the fat that hides those muscles (especially if it squeezes around your internal organs) is associated with an increased risk of diabetes, heart disease, and other health problems.

To help you firm your abs and reap all of these health benefits, top fitness researchers tested more than a dozen tummy-toning exercises in the lab and, using sensitive equipment to analyze muscle activity, came out with the definitive answers on which ones work best. In this chapter, we bring you those exercises. No more wasted time and effort. Just results—in as little as 14 days!

The Science of Ab Exercises

To come up with the very best tummy-toning moves, researchers at San Diego State University asked 31 people—both occasional and daily exercisers ages 20 to 45—to perform 13 exercises that target the midsection while the researchers measured the work of the abdominals. (They looked at both the rectus abdominis, which runs the length of your torso and is the "workhorse," and the obliques, or side-lying muscles that rotate your body and stabilize the pelvis.) Then they compared how each exercise stacked up against the traditional crunch.

The two top-ranking exercises: The bicycle maneuver and the captain's chair were up to 2½ times more effective at working the obliques and at least 50% better at strengthening the rectus abdominis compared with the traditional crunch.

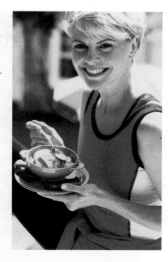

Diet and Exercise: Still Key

We're not going to kid you: To get abs worthy of admiring glances, you still need to eat a sensible diet and do regular aerobic activity at least 5 days a week. Otherwise, no amount of crunches will help you trim the layer of fat that may be hiding the fabulous abdominal muscles you'll be building with this program.

Other winning moves: The long arm crunch and the crunch on an exercise ball (also known as a Swiss ball) both isolate the ab muscles specifically, rather than relying on the hip flexors at the front of the hip to help out with the move (as is the case with traditional crunches), says lead researcher Peter Francis, PhD, director of the biomechanics lab at San Diego State University. Crunches on an exercise ball also force your abs to work overtime just to stabilize you atop the ball and enable you to train in a greater, more natural range of motion.

Based on the findings of this study, we picked the top six exercises for our belly-flattening plan, arranging them in three programs from beginner to advanced.

Prevention's Best Belly-Flattening Program

Here they are: The best abdominal exercises science has to offer. Pick one of our three customized programs to suit your experience. To keep your back strong and in balance with the front and side torso muscles, we've included a back extension. And since some of the exercises require hip motion, we've added a hip stretch, so your hip flexors don't become tight.

Getting started: Before you try any of the plans, be sure you've mastered the basic crunch (see "Make Every Crunch Count" on p. 69).

Repetitions: Perform 10 to 12 repetitions of each exercise (when just starting out, do only as many as you can, even if it's just four or five); this equals one set. Move slowly: 2 or 3 seconds up, hold 1 second, and 2 or 3 seconds down.

Choose Your Program

	Exercises (do 1 set of each per session)	Frequency
BEGINNER	Reverse Crunch	3 days/week
	Vertical Leg Crunch	
	Long Arm Crunch	
	Back Extension	
EXPERIENCED	Bicycle Maneuver	3–5 days/week
	Captain's Chair	
	Crunch on an Exercise Ball	
	Back Extension	
	Hip Flexor Stretch	
ADVANCED	Bicycle Maneuver	5 days/week
	Captain's Chair	
	Reverse Crunch	
	Crunch on an Exercise Ball	
	Vertical Leg Crunch	
	Long Arm Crunch	
	Back Extension	
	Hip Flexor Stretch	

If you feel back pain with any of these exercises, stop, try another exercise, and consult your doctor.

BICYCLE MANEUVER

Lie with your lower back pressed into the floor and your hands clasped lightly behind your head. Bend your knees to about a 45-degree angle from the floor. Simultaneously, lift your shoulders off the floor, and bring your left knee to your right elbow, while straightening your right leg. Then using a bicycle pedaling motion, straighten your left knee while bringing the right knee in toward the left elbow. Extend your legs out only as far as is comfortable without arching your back. Continue alternating, keeping the movement slow and controlled.

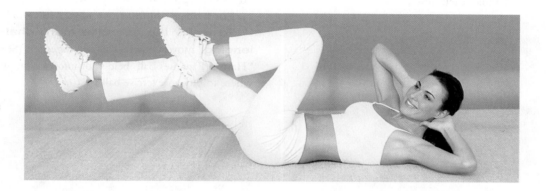

CAPTAIN'S CHAIR

Sit up straight in a firm, armless chair. Grab the chair's edges just in front of your hips. While supporting yourself with your hands, slowly draw your knees up toward your chest, keeping your lower back pressed against the chair. Hold, then slowly lower.

To make this move more challenging, start by using your arms to hold yourself suspended in the air.

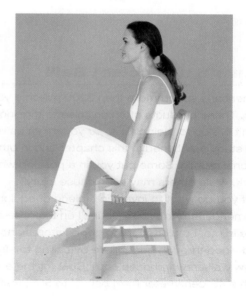

REVERSE CRUNCH

Lie on the floor with your arms at your sides, feet off the floor, and hips and knees bent at 90-degree angles. Slowly contract your abs, and press your back into the floor, tilting your pelvis and lifting your hips 2 to 4" off the floor. Keep your upper body relaxed. Hold, then slowly lower.

CRUNCH ON AN EXERCISE BALL

Lie back on an exercise ball so that the ball is supporting your lower back, with your knees bent, and your feet flat on the floor. Place your hands loosely behind your head. Slowly raise your shoulders to no more than 45 degrees up from horizontal. Hold, then slowly lower.

For better balance, spread your feet wider.

To make the exercise more challenging, move your feet closer together. (See "Have a (Exercise) Ball" below for information on where to buy an exercise ball.)

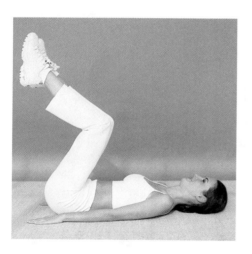

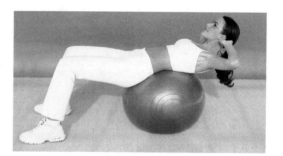

Have a (Exercise) Ball!

Americans spend more than $200 million a year on abdominal devices in a quest for flat, firm abs. These products often promise to trim inches in "just minutes a day." The fact is, most don't live up to their claims, so you might as well save your money. The products tested in the study mentioned in this chapter and in other research all rated less effective than the traditional crunch. Some put you in a position where your abdominal muscles barely do any work, while others may even cause injury.

If you *do* want to invest in a piece of equipment, choose the highly rated exercise ball, recommends the American Council on Exercise in San Diego. Inflatable exercise balls are available in most major sporting goods stores and cost around $30. Or you can buy a ball, pump, and video through our affiliate by calling toll-free (888) 972-9255, or online by visiting www.walkerswarehouse.com. Cost for the entire package is $35. (If you're under 5' tall, go with a 45-centimeter [cm] ball; 5' to 5'7", try the 55-cm size; over 5'7", buy a 65-cm ball.)

DO JUST ONE THING!

Make Every Crunch Count

There's nothing wrong with the traditional crunch. In fact, mastering proper technique with this basic exercise is one of the most effective things you can do to strengthen your abdominals, since so many exercises are based on this single move. Here's how to make sure your form is good (and effective!):

- ▶ Go slow.

- ▶ Focus on using just your abdominal muscles.

- ▶ Don't pull on your neck or tuck your chin.

- ▶ Lift only until your shoulder blades clear the floor.

- ▶ Press your lower back firmly into the floor.

- ▶ Pause at the top position for at least 1 second.

According to *Prevention* advisor Wayne L. Westcott, PhD, fitness research director for the South Shore YMCA in Quincy, MA, the last two steps are often neglected, but are crucial to fully activate the abdominal muscles.

VERTICAL LEG CRUNCH

Lie on your back, and extend your legs straight up in the air, feet crossed at the ankles, with a slight bend in the knees. Place your hands loosely behind your head. Contract your abdominals, and slowly raise your head, shoulders, and upper back about 30 degrees, or 3 to 5", off the floor. Hold, then slowly lower. Keep your legs still. (This move can also be done with your lower legs resting on a chair or bed.)

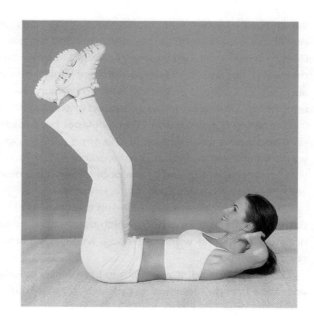

LONG ARM CRUNCH

Lie on your back with your knees bent and your feet flat on the floor. Extend your arms overhead. Slowly raise your arms, head, shoulders, and upper back about 45 degrees off the floor. Hold, then slowly lower. Keep your arms straight, by your ears, and in line with your head. Do not throw them forward to help you.

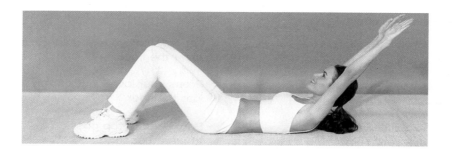

"I Tone My Whole Body in the Pool!"

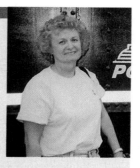

When Nancy Moffett first discovered that she had post-polio syndrome (which causes extreme fatigue and back and leg pain), her active lifestyle ground to a halt. "I knew I needed to keep exercising to maintain my health, but walks and home aerobics wiped me out. On my doctor's suggestion, I started swimming laps. To my surprise, I woke up the day after my first session feeling energized instead of achy!" she explains.

Swimming burns 476 to 680 calories per hour (based on a 150-lb person) and works the entire body: the arms and legs are obvious beneficiaries of the activity, but your abdominals also get a great workout when you turn your body to take a breath and when you flip around at the end of the pool to begin the next lap. It's also easy on the joints and not very likely to cause workout-related injuries.

Today, Nancy alternates between the crawl and breaststroke coupled with a dolphin kick (keeping both legs together), which doesn't tire her legs as much. "I now regularly swim a nonstop 30-minute workout twice a week, and I strength train another two times a week," says Nancy.

Getting started. If you'd like to burn some calories without getting all hot and sweaty, call your local college, health club, or YMCA for information about pool use and swimming classes.

BACK EXTENSION

Note: If you have lower-back pain, consult your doctor before doing this exercise. Lie on your belly, keeping your hips and pelvis flat. With your hands under your chin, contract your lower back muscles, and lift your chest about 30 degrees, or 3 to 5", off the floor. Hold, then slowly lower.

To make the exercise easier, rest your arms by your sides, palms facing up.
To make the exercise more challenging, extend your arms straight overhead.

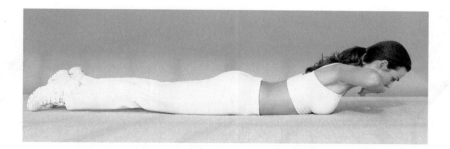

HIP FLEXOR STRETCH

Stand with your feet a few inches apart, then move one leg about 1 to 2' forward. Bend your knees, making sure your front knee is directly over the ankle, and your back heel is off the floor. Hold in your belly, and tuck your butt by tilting your pelvis. You should feel the stretch at the front of your hips. Hold for 15 to 60 seconds, then switch legs.

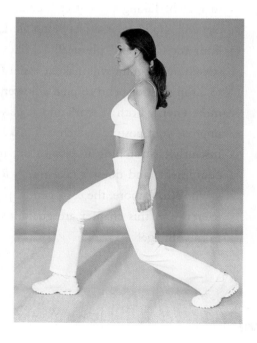

CHAPTER 10

Seven Easy Feel-Good Stretches

Double your energy, ease pain, and look fabulous!

You probably already know that stretching is important for improving your flexibility and preventing soreness after exercise, but those aren't the only reasons to stretch! Taking a few stretch breaks throughout the day will also make you feel better all day, every day—both mentally and physically! Following a regular stretching program will make it easier for you to reach to a top shelf or bend to pick a flower, it will give you more energy both at work and at play, and it will help improve your posture (which will make you look slimmer instantly!). Stretching is easy to do, requires no special equipment, and doesn't take much longer than a good yawn. What's more, the easy, gentle, pleasurable stretching exercises in this chapter are guaranteed to subtract years from your age!

Flexibility is the Fountain of Youth.

How Stretching Makes You Younger

Starting in your 30s, your body's connective tissues—muscles, tendons, and ligaments—start to shorten and tighten, losing elasticity, says Marilyn Moffat, PhD, PT, past president of the American Physical Therapy Association and professor of physical therapy at New York University in New York City. Even more than aging, poor posture causes tightening and impedes bloodflow. Over time, this can create a buildup of calcifications (those hard knots you may have in your upper back), plus a hunched look and restricted movement.

But despite the damage you've already done, flexibility *can* be regained by stretching regularly—and improvement can be seen within weeks. When you stretch, you lengthen the muscles and tendons, increasing flexibility. When a muscle is flexible, it enables the joint to completely flex, extend, and move in multiple directions (known as range of motion)—whether it's to throw a baseball or turn a car's steering wheel.

Stretching Can Help You...

- ▶ Ease into an exercise program
- ▶ Prevent soreness after exercise
- ▶ Maximize strength gains
- ▶ Increase flexibility and range of motion
- ▶ Relieve back, joint, and muscle pain
- ▶ Enhance body awareness
- ▶ Improve coordination
- ▶ Perform daily tasks more easily
- ▶ Sharpen mental focus
- ▶ Relax, de-stress, and boost your mood
- ▶ Improve your circulation
- ▶ Reduce stiffness
- ▶ Boost your energy level
- ▶ Improve your posture

Enhanced flexibility and range of movement also affect your life in ways you don't realize. In one study, participants age 60 and older increased their everyday walking speed by simply stretching regularly—nothing else.

DO JUST ONE THING!

Improve Your Form

To maximize the benefits of stretching (and to prevent injuries), familiarize yourself with these "10 Commandments of Stretching" today.

1. Follow a program that is specific to your activities and needs. (See "Your Customized Stretching Routine" on p. 74.)

2. Stretch regularly, at least three times a week.

3. Warm up before stretching (either with a workout or a few minutes of walking).

4. Stretch only to the point where you feel tension in the belly of the muscle, not pain in the joint.

5. Hold each stretch for 15 to 60 seconds.

6. Do each stretch 2 to 4 times.

7. Stay relaxed as you stretch.

8. Breathe throughout the stretch.

9. Progress in a slow, controlled manner.

10. Don't bounce.

Your Customized Stretching Routine

On the following pages, you'll find a whole day's worth of stretches recommended by Jo Fasen, PT, orthopedic clinical specialist at the Rehabilitation Institute of Chicago's Center for Spine, Sports, and Occupational Rehabilitation. You can do them all for a stress-relieving, invigorating routine, or do individual stretches for specific problems. If you don't see improvement after a month of consistent stretching, or you still have pain, see a physical therapist.

Choose Your Program

If you're . . .	Do these stretches . . . *	Because you need to . . .
At a desk all day or an avid cyclist	The Morning Stress Reliever (10 AM) The Evening Energizer (8 PM) The Bedtime Body Soother (10 PM)	Do extension exercises that open the chest and the front of the hips and that lengthen the back of the thighs and spine.
On your feet all day or a walker or runner	The Morning Energizer (7 AM) The After-Work Revitalizer (6 PM) The Bedtime Body Soother (10 PM)	Relieve the muscles that have been used all day: the calves, the front of the thighs, and the back.
A new mother	The Morning Stress Reliever (10 AM) The Afternoon Energizer (3 PM) The Bedtime Body Soother (10 PM)	Reverse the rounded posture that can be caused by breastfeeding and carrying your baby.
A woman age 60 or older	The Morning Stress Reliever (10 AM) The After-Lunch Stretch (1 PM) The Bedtime Body Soother (10 PM)	Stretch your chest (to prevent hunching over) and your hips and calves (to optimize walking and balance).

*Perform each stretch 2 to 4 times, and do each group of stretches at least 3 times per week.

THE MORNING ENERGIZER (7AM)
BACK, SHOULDERS, AND ABS

Benefits: Relieves back pain and helps energize you

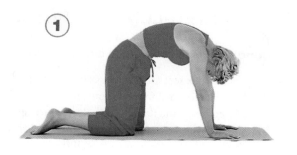

Kneel on your hands and knees with your head, neck, and back in alignment and your back flat. Keeping your shoulders relaxed, lower your chin toward your chest, pull in your belly, and round your back, like a cat arching its back (photo 1). You'll feel this stretch throughout your back and shoulders.

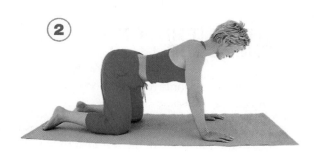

Hold, then slowly return to the starting position. Next, arch your back in the opposite direction, creating an inward curve with your butt lifted toward the ceiling and your head looking up just slightly (photo 2). You'll feel the stretch throughout your back and abdominals. Hold, then repeat the sequence.

THE MORNING STRESS RELIEVER (10 AM)
CHEST, SHOULDERS, AND UPPER BACK

Benefits: Reduces stress and improves mental focus

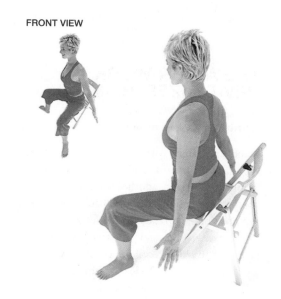

FRONT VIEW

Sit on the edge of a chair with your pelvis tilted slightly forward and your legs spread as wide as comfortable. Slide your chin back so that your ears align over your shoulders. Lift your chest, and squeeze your shoulder blades together and down away from your ears. Reach both arms wide and slightly behind you. Your palms should be facing forward, fingers spread. Don't arch your lower back. You'll feel the stretch in your chest, shoulders, and upper back. Hold, then repeat.

THE AFTER-LUNCH STRETCH (1 PM)
HIPS

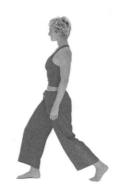

Benefits: Prevents soreness after a lunchtime walk and also reduces hip pain

Stand with your feet a few inches apart, then move one leg about 1 to 2' forward. Bend your knees, making sure your front knee is directly over the ankle. Your back heel will come off the floor. Keep your posture upright as you tuck in your abdomen and butt and tilt your pelvis. Hold. You'll feel this stretch at the front of your hip area. Switch legs, and repeat to stretch the other hip.

THE AFTERNOON ENERGIZER (3 PM)
NECK

BACK VIEW

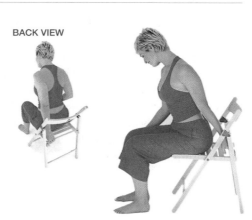

Benefits: Prevents an afternoon slump and eases neck pain

While sitting in a chair, hook your left hand, palm facing you, on the back of the seat next to your left buttock. Hold on as you lean forward. Keep your shoulders back, and drop your right ear toward your right shoulder. Then roll your chin forward, and hold. You'll feel this stretch at the left side of your neck. Switch hands, and repeat to stretch the right side of your neck.

THE AFTER-WORK REVITALIZER (6 PM)
ABS, SIDES, AND BACK

Benefits: Calms anxiety

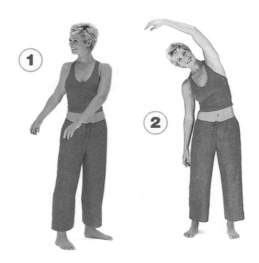

Stand up straight with your feet shoulder-width apart, hips facing forward, and abs tight. Gently twist your trunk to the right, and hold (photo 1). You'll feel this stretch in your abs, sides, and back. Return to the starting position, and repeat to the left side.

Next, gently lean to the right as you reach your left arm up toward the ceiling; curve it slightly overhead, palm down (photo 2). Keep your shoulders down and relaxed. Hold, then repeat to the left side. You'll feel this stretch along the sides of your torso.

THE EVENING ENERGIZER (8 PM)

BUTT, THIGHS, CHEST, UPPER BACK, SHOULDERS, AND ABS

Benefits: Improves posture and muscle tone—
great to do before going out for the evening

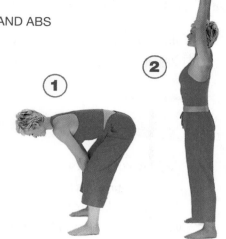

Stand with your feet shoulder-width apart and your abs tight.
Keeping your back straight, bend at the hips and knees,
reaching your hands through your legs, if comfortable (photo
1). Hold. *Caution:* Don't do this if you have back pain. You'll
feel this stretch in your butt and thighs.

Next, use your hips to straighten up, reaching your
arms overhead and slightly behind you (photo 2). Hold.
Don't arch your back. You'll feel this stretch in your chest,
upper back, shoulders, and abs. Repeat the entire sequence.

THE BEDTIME BODY SOOTHER (10 PM)

SHOULDERS, BACK, CHEST, AND HIPS

Benefits: Relax, prepare for sleep, and ease shoulder pain

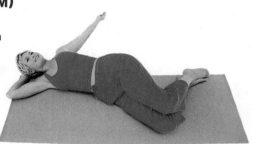

Lie on the floor on your right side with your right arm bent
underneath your head. Bend both legs so you're comfortable.
Imagine that you're lying on a big clock. Extend your left
arm in front of you on the floor as if it's a clock hand pointing to 9 o'clock. Slowly rotate your arm toward 12 o'clock.
As you hit 1 o'clock, you'll start to roll back, but keep your
hips and legs where they are. Keeping your arm on the floor, rotate it through all the numbers on the
clock (your palm will flip up momentarily behind you), over your hips, and back to the starting position.
You'll feel this stretch in your shoulders and upper back, then chest and middle back, and finally hips and
lower back. Switch sides, and repeat with the other arm.

Stretch after Exercise

If you are using the stretches in this chapter to improve flexibility when you work out, be sure
to do them *after* your exercise routine, not before. Your muscles will be warm after you've
worked out, making them more pliable. This is when you'll gain the biggest improvements in
flexibility. Stretching when muscles are warm also decreases the likelihood of injury.

Your Get-Fit-Faster Planner

Simplify your workout, and maximize your motivation with this handy checklist!

Two of the best ways to encourage yourself to stick with an exercise program are to chart your progress and to reward yourself for a job well done. That's why we've provided this handy planner for doing just that. You may want to photocopy it several times, so you can use it over and over again!

Note: We've listed "walking workout," "ab exercises," and "stretching exercises" every day because *you* get to choose when you want to do them; however, be sure to check the workout plans in Chapters 8, 9, and 10 to see exactly how many days you need to schedule for each. (You can use a highlighter to mark the days you plan on doing each type of exercise.)

Goals and Rewards

Before you get started, jot down what you plan to do in the next 4 weeks, and note a healthy reward you'll give yourself each Sunday after you've met those goals. Some ideas: a pedicure, a new CD, some workout gear, a massage, a book, a workout tape, or a day trip to a nearby tourist spot.

WEEK 1	Goals:
	Reward:
WEEK 2	Goals:
	Reward:
WEEK 3	Goals:
	Reward:
WEEK 4	Goals:
	Reward:

		WEEK 1	WEEK 2	WEEK 3	WEEK 4
MONDAY	Walking workout p. 58				
	Chest: Dumbell Press p. 51				
	Back: Two-Arm Row p. 51				
	Ab exercises p. 66				
	Stretching exercises p.74				
TUESDAY	Walking workout p. 58				
	Shoulders: Lateral Raise p. 52				
	Abdominals: Crunch p. 52				
	Ab exercises p. 66				
	Stretching exercises p. 74				
WEDNESDAY	Walking workout p. 58				
	Triceps: Lying Kickback p. 53				
	Biceps: Standing Curl p. 53				
	Ab exercises p. 66				
	Stretching exercises p. 74				
THURSDAY	Walking workout p. 58				
	Hamstrings: Leg Lift p. 54				
	Quadriceps: Squat p. 54				
	Ab exercises p. 66				
	Stretching exercises p. 74				
FRIDAY	Walking workout p. 58				
	Calves: Standing Raise p. 55				
	Butt: Kick-Up p. 55				
	Ab exercises p. 66				
	Stretching exercises p. 74				
SATURDAY	Walking workout p. 58				
	Inner-Thigh Leg Raise p. 56				
	Outer Thigh: Doggie p. 56				
	Ab exercises p. 66				
	Stretching exercises p. 74				
SUNDAY	Walking workout p. 58				
	Ab exercises p. 66				
	Stretching exercises p. 74				

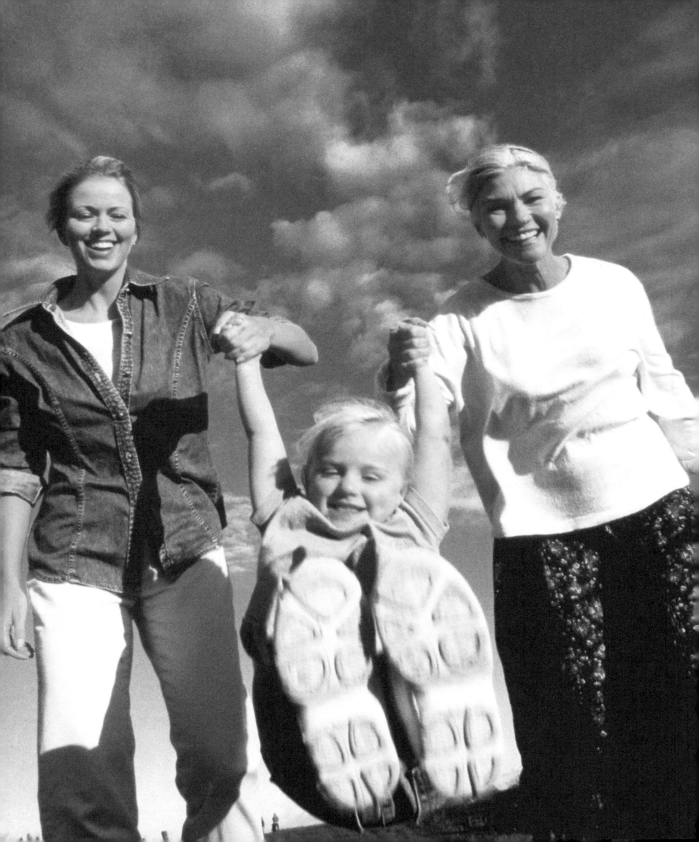

PART **THREE**

Safeguard Your Health

CHAPTER 11

The Lowdown on Genetic Risks

Powerful steps you can take if your genetics put you at risk for cancer, heart disease, or diabetes

If your mom was diagnosed with cancer, heart disease, diabetes, or some other health problem with a genetic link, you may wonder if you'll get the same diagnosis one day. "When it comes to breast cancer in particular, many women look at their mother's experience" for a preview of their own, says Michael Thun, MD, an epidemiological researcher with the Atlanta-based American Cancer Society (ACS). "But if that's all you look at, you're missing more than half the picture."

For starters, you're missing your father's 50% contribution to your genetic makeup. And you're overlooking the role that lifestyle plays. Whether you smoke, eat your fruits and vegetables, exercise regularly, and get screening tests all affect your odds of developing a variety of serious

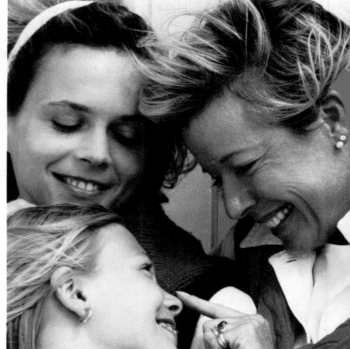

Learn your risks so *all* can avoid them!

health problems. Here's the lowdown on how a family history of certain diseases can affect you—and what to do to stay on the good side of the statistics.

‖ Breast Cancer

If you have a distant relative (such as a cousin or great-grandmother) with breast cancer, you have a slightly higher risk than the average 1-in-8 lifetime risk of getting the disease.

If you have a parent, sibling, or child with breast cancer (men can get the disease too), your risk could be double. The risk is even higher if that relative was diagnosed before age 50. And having two first-degree relatives can boost the odds as much as threefold.

The Genetic Tie-In

In some families, the culprit is a mutation or glitch in the genes known as BRCA1 and BRCA2, which you can inherit from your mom or dad and that may also increase your risk of ovarian cancer. Of the 1 in 200 women with a mutation, about 50 to 80% will develop breast cancer.

Improve Your Odds

Even if you don't have a family history, there's some evidence that staying close to your ideal weight, exercising, eating lots of produce and little fat, and having no more than one alcoholic drink a day may help you avoid breast cancer, says Debbie Saslow, PhD, the ACS's director of breast and gynecologic cancers. (See Chapter 13 for more tips on reducing your risk for breast cancer.) If you have a strong family history of breast cancer (more than one close relative with it), you should also follow this advice.

1-MINUTE *FAT BLASTER*

Schedule a Genetic Checkup

A genetic counselor can help you evaluate your risk of cancer, outline the pros and cons of genetic testing, and develop a plan to help you minimize that risk.

To find one in your area, call the National Society of Genetic Counselors at (610) 872-7608 (press 7 for the consumer line). Or visit their Web site at www.nsgc.org. Some, but not all, insurance companies will pay for counseling and testing, so call yours for details.

See a genetic counselor. A counselor can analyze your risk and help you decide whether to get tested for BRCA mutations.

Step up the screening tests. In addition to doing a monthly breast self-exam that everyone should start at age 20, ask your doctor about these screening tests, which can help detect cancer early, when it's most treatable.

Clinical breast exam. You should have one of these as often as every 6 months, starting at age 20, if you have known mutations in the BRCA genes or a strong family history.

Mammogram. Some experts recommend yearly mammograms 10 years before the youngest age of diagnosis in your family. Many advise women with BRCA mutations to start getting screened between ages 25 and 35.

Breast ultrasonography and MRI. These tests may help detect breast cancer in the denser breasts of younger women.

Talk about other options. The drug tamoxifen may lower breast cancer risk by as much as 50% in women at high risk. Surgery to remove the breasts can also lower risk substantially, as can surgical removal of the ovaries, but these are more drastic steps.

Ask about ductal lavage. This recently approved procedure involves analyzing cells from the breast milk ducts (where more than 90% of breast cancers start) for abnormalities associated with cancer. The results can help women further evaluate their risk and decide whether to use drugs such as tamoxifen, Dr. Saslow explains.

‖ Colon Cancer

If you have a parent, sibling, or child with colon cancer, you have a somewhat higher lifetime risk—about 6%—compared with

the average American's risk of 2%. If your relative was diagnosed before age 45, your risk rises to 10%. It's about 17% for women who have two first-degree relatives with the disease.

If you have a family history of ovarian, uterine, or breast cancer, you are also at higher risk for colon cancer.

The Genetic Tie-In

Those at very high risk for colon cancer are people with one of two syndromes caused by genetic mutations: familial adenomatous polyposis syndrome (FAP) or hereditary nonpolyposis colon cancer (HNPCC). People with FAP develop hundreds of precancerous polyps or growths in their colons and are virtually guaranteed to get col-

---

DO JUST ONE THING!
Take *the* Healthiest Step

Smoking-related illnesses among women have reached epidemic proportions, killing 3 million American women in the past 2 decades, according to the shocking "Women and Smoking: A Report of the Surgeon General—2001."

"Lung cancer is now the leading cancer killer among women, exceeding breast cancer," says Corinne Husten, MD, MPH, a medical officer at the Atlanta-based Centers for Disease Control and Prevention. But that's not all: A new study tracking 902 heart attack patients suggests that smoking just one cigarette could trigger a repeat attack. "Not smoking, or quitting if you smoke cigarettes now, is the number one thing you can do for your health," Dr. Husten says. Here's some of what smoking does to your body.

Smoking boosts the risk of

▶ lung, bladder, pancreatic, cervical, and other cancers

▶ emphysema

▶ chronic obstructive pulmonary disease

Smoking has been linked to

▶ infertility

▶ miscarriage

▶ low birth weight deliveries

▶ more severe menopause symptoms

▶ stroke

▶ repeat heart attacks

orectal cancer unless they have their colons removed in early adulthood, explains Durado Brooks, MD, the ACS's director for colon cancer. Those with HNPCC run a 70 to 80% chance of developing colon cancer.

Improve Your Odds

Once again, there are things everyone should do to lower their risk of colon cancer. "Eating a low-fat, low-meat, high-vegetable diet, getting regular physical activity, and avoiding obesity and cigarettes are all good ideas," Dr. Brooks says. There's also some evidence that calcium supplements and about 400 micrograms (mcg) of folic acid daily may lower risk. (See Chapter 13 for more tips for reducing your risk for this cancer.) If you're at increased risk of colon cancer, you should also do the following.

Find out whether testing is for you. If one relative or more has FAP, consider counseling and genetic testing. You should also consider counseling and testing for the HNPCC mutation if your family includes at least three people with colon cancer (including two first-degree relatives), people from at least two generations with the disease, and at least one person diagnosed before turning 50.

Step up screening. *Prevention* recommends colorectal screening for most people starting at age 50, but you should start earlier if you meet any of the following criteria.

You're at increased risk. Starting at age 40, or 10 years before the earliest case in your immediate family, get a colonoscopy every 5 to 10 years.

A family history of FAP. Start getting regular endoscopies and colonoscopies at puberty.

A family history of HNPCC. Schedule a colonoscopy at age 21, and repeat it every 1 to 2

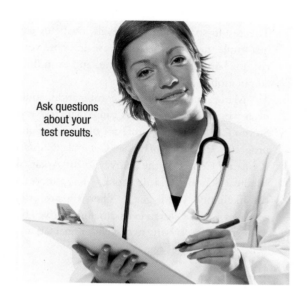

Ask questions about your test results.

years until age 40, when you should start getting an annual colonoscopy.

Ask your doctor about celecoxib. In a recent study, people with FAP who took the drug celecoxib developed fewer precancerous colorectal polyps than those not taking the drug. Researchers are trying to determine whether it can lower the risk of other hereditary colon cancers.

‖ Type 2 Diabetes

If you have a parent or sibling with the disease, your lifetime risk is about 38%.

If both parents have diabetes, your odds could soar as high as 80%.

The Genetic Tie-In

In type 2 diabetes (the most common form), your body stops responding to insulin, the hormone that delivers sugar into cells, and it does not produce enough insulin to overcome this problem.

The result: soaring insulin levels. Diabetes can quadruple the risk of heart disease and raise your risk for blindness, kidney failure, and even limb amputation.

Many genes, singly or in combination, could be at work. "But genes don't cause diabetes," says Steven C. Elbein, MD, professor of medicine and program director of the General Clinical Research Center at the University of Arkansas Medical School in Little Rock. "They increase the likelihood you'll get it. There's a powerful interplay between lifestyle risk (being overweight, not exercising, carrying excess abdominal fat) and genetic risk."

Improve Your Odds

Despite your family history, you can take simple steps every day that dramatically reduce your risks. These measures can also keep hidden diabetes genes turned off. Here's what Dr. Elbein suggests.

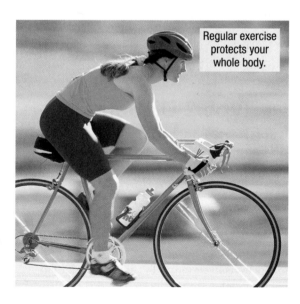

Regular exercise protects your whole body.

Know your numbers. Diabetes and early diabetes (known as impaired fasting glucose) are easy to detect with a simple blood check called a fasting plasma glucose test (performed after an 8- to 12-hour fast). A reading of 109 mg/dl or less is normal; 110 to 125 mg/dl indicates impaired fasting glucose; 126 or higher is a sign of full-blown diabetes.

If results are normal, repeat the test once a year. If you have early diabetes, repeat it every 6 months. If you have full-blown diabetes, discuss testing with your doctor.

Drop a few pounds. Among the 3,324 participants in the Diabetes Prevention Program (DPP) study, those who lost just 5 to 7% of their body weight (usually by exercising half an hour a day and eating a healthy diet) reduced their risk of diabetes by 58%.

Remake your plate. DPP participants also ate more fruit, veggies, and whole grains, and less fat (less than 30% of daily calories). This strategy not only helps you lose weight, but it may help trim abdominal fat, which is a potent risk for diabetes, Dr. Elbein says.

Get moving. The DPP study aimed for just 30 minutes of exercise, five times a week, and it got big results. Moderate exercise (walking, biking, playing tennis) is enough to improve your odds, though more is better.

‖ Heart Disease

If you have one parent, sibling, or child who had a heart attack by age 55 in men or 65 in women, your risk is 3 to 4 times higher than that of the general population.

If you have two siblings or other first-degree relatives who meet the

Switch Snacks, Save Your Heart

New findings from the landmark Nurses' Health Study confirm mounting evidence that filling up on refined carbohydrates can increase heart disease risk, especially in postmenopausal women.

When Harvard researchers tested blood samples from 280 healthy female nurses ages 45 to 70, they found that those with the highest glycemic load—a measure of carbohydrate intake and its ability to raise blood sugar and insulin—had 10% less HDL cholesterol, the kind that helps keep arteries clear. What's more, their triglyceride levels were 76% higher, which raised heart disease risk significantly.

The better way to control weight and be good to your heart? "Instead of simply replacing fat with carbohydrates, improve the quality of the carbohydrates you consume, and incorporate healthy fats such as olive oil, fatty fish, and nuts," says Simin Liu, MD, assistant professor of medicine at Harvard Medical School. Here are a few healthy switches to get you started.

GOOD-CARB MUNCHIES

Instead of these	Have these
Graham crackers	Oatmeal cookie
Low-fat cookies	Half a peanut butter and jelly sandwich on oat bran bread
Baked chips and salsa	Small stone-ground whole wheat pita with hummus
Vanilla wafers	Canned peaches or apricots in natural juice
Bagel	Banana bread
Jelly beans	2 tablespoons peanuts

above criteria, your risk of an early heart attack is 12 times that of the general population.

The Genetic Tie-In

One of the most common genetic defects is familial hypercholesterolemia (FH). The half-million-plus Americans with FH have sky-high levels of total cholesterol (300 to 500), near-normal triglyceride levels, and a family history of early heart attacks: between 40 and 55 for men, 50 and 65 for women. The danger: FH increases heart attack risk 20 to 25 times, and it can lead to heart attack as early as age 20!

Another widespread but under-recognized hereditary threat is metabolic syndrome. Also called syndrome X, this lethal, often-inherited combination of abdominal fat (a waist measuring more than 35 inches for women, 40 inches for men), triglycerides higher than 150 mg/dl, low levels of HDLs (less than 50 for women, less than 40 for men), and early (or full-blown) diabetes raises heart attack risk even if total cholesterol is normal.

Researchers have identified dozens of genes that may play a role in heart attack, high cholesterol, and high blood pressure. "We believe that even mildly elevated cholesterol can be hereditary," explains Paul Hopkins, MD, associate professor of internal medicine at the University of Utah in Salt Lake City and a codirector of the university's Cardiovascular Genetics Research Clinic. "But in many cases, these genes simply make you more susceptible to cardiovascular problems."

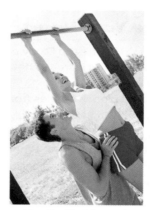

A healthy lifestyle equals a healthier future!

Improve Your Odds

As with many other serious health conditions, if you control your weight, eat healthfully, and exercise regularly, you can minimize your risk. Once you've figured out your own family history, these steps can help too.

Share your history with your doctor. If you find evidence of early heart attack, a pattern of high cholesterol and/or high trigylceride levels, or a history of diabetes in your family tree, tell your doctor. Map out a strategy for regular cholesterol, triglyceride, and blood sugar checks, as well as blood pressure monitoring.

Ask about drugs if you have FH. Ask your doctor about cholesterol-lowering statins, bile acid sequestrants, and niacin therapy. "Even without other risk factors for heart attacks, and with the best of health habits, heart attacks will almost certainly occur in people with FH if cholesterol levels are not lowered," Dr. Hopkins says. Lifestyle efforts are usually not enough.

Live healthy. The same exercise and eating strategies that will help reduce your diabetes risk can lower your heart attack risk as well. If your parents or siblings had heart disease later in life, start with a lifestyle strategy; add medications if your cholesterol or blood pressure readings still need a nudge downward.

Aim for these numbers. A panel of top heart experts suggests that you aim for these optimal cholesterol levels if you have a genetic risk for heart disease:

▶ LDL less than 100
▶ HDL more than 40
▶ Total cholesterol less than 200
▶ Blood pressure less than 140/90 (Some evidence suggests that less than 130/85 is more protective.)

Watch your blood sugar. Even early diabetes (slightly elevated blood sugar) significantly raises heart disease risk. Get checked now, and talk with your doctor about a treatment and testing strategy.

CHAPTER 12

All Your Cholesterol Questions Answered

Why high cholesterol can kill you—and how to bring those numbers down *now*

When people start talking about cholesterol, all those numbers and acronyms—HDL, LDL—are enough to make your eyes glaze over. But cholesterol is something that you *should* pay attention to, because having high cholesterol increases your risk of developing cardiovascular disease, the number one cause of death in the US today. And bringing your cholesterol levels down—which, by the way, is very doable—really does make a difference. In fact, for every 1% drop in your total cholesterol, you reduce your heart attack risk by 1 to 2%.

But just what is high cholesterol, and what does it have to do with your heart? Well, that's what this chapter is here to help you understand—in plain, simple English. On the pages that follow, you'll find out once and for all

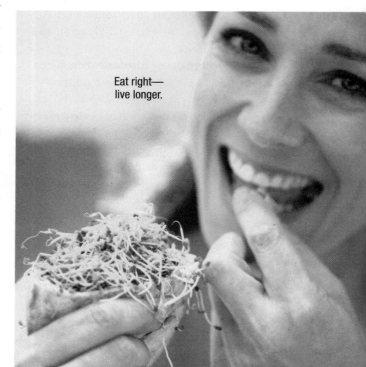

Eat right—
live longer.

what all those numbers mean (it's simpler than it may seem), and then we'll tell you which healthy habits can reduce your cholesterol for good. And the next time a friend's eyes start to glaze over when you start to talk about cholesterol, you can let them take a look at this chapter too!

What Does Cholesterol Do?

Cholesterol is a fatty substance made by your liver. And despite its bad reputation, you actually *do* need it. It helps to form cell membranes and some of your hormones too. So where is the problem? Well, your body makes all the cholesterol it needs. So when you eat foods that are high in saturated fat, which triggers your liver to churn out *more* cholesterol, you're left with an abundance of cholesterol that's got nowhere to go. That excess cholesterol builds up in your arteries, blocks bloodflow, and, if left untreated, can set the stage for heart attack and stroke. The higher the amount of excess cholesterol, the worse the health risk.

The two types of cholesterol: When you hear people talk about cholesterol, you've likely heard two acronyms—LDLs and HDLs. These are actually the two types of cholesterol—low-density lipoproteins (LDLs) and high-density lipoproteins (HDLs). Lipoproteins are combinations of fat and protein made by your body. It's

their job to deliver other fats—which don't dissolve in blood—to your cells.

What is LDL? Often called the "bad" cholesterol, LDL carries most of the cholesterol in the blood. When there's too much LDL, it can combine with other substances to form a plaque in your arteries, which can stick to the artery walls. If a blood clot develops in the vicinity of a plaque formation, it can further restrict bloodflow, possibly leading to a heart attack or stroke. Experts now think that the lower your LDL level, the better.

What is HDL? HDL is known as the "good" cholesterol. It carries about one-fourth to one-third of the cholesterol in the blood, transporting it from different organs to the liver for disposal from the body. HDL may also pick up cholesterol deposited in your arteries and move it on out, preventing it from building up in your arteries.

Am I at Risk?

The same risk factors that make you susceptible for heart disease also make you susceptible to high blood cholesterol. Some you can't control, some you can. Here are the top risk factors for high cholesterol.

Your age. The likelihood of high cholesterol (and heart attack) increases with age. The vast majority of people who die from heart disease are age 65 or older.

Your family history. Genes help determine how your body handles LDL cholesterol.

You can bring down your cholesterol 20 to 50% simply by eating right and exercising.

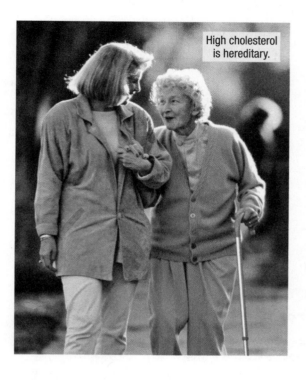

High cholesterol is hereditary.

You're more likely to have high cholesterol if your parents had heart disease.

Your gender. Women have a lower risk for heart attacks than men, but don't let that lull you into complacency. Women over age 65 who have heart attacks are twice as likely as men to die from them.

Your lifestyle. To keep your cholesterol levels as healthy as possible, cut back on fat, exercise regularly, don't smoke, maintain a healthy weight, and take cholesterol-lowering medications if your doctor prescribes them. (See "How Can I Lower My Cholesterol?" on p. 93 for tips on modifying your lifestyle to bring your cholesterol down or prevent it from rising in the first place.)

Should I Get Tested?

The National Cholesterol Education Program, an initiative of the National Heart, Lung, and Blood Institute, advises the following.

Everyone age 20 and older should get their cholesterol checked once every 5 years.

Women over 55 (and men over 45) should ask their doctor if they should be tested more frequently than every 5 years, since cholesterol levels tend to rise with age.

If you are diagnosed with high cholesterol, or if you're in a high risk group, your doctor will likely want to have you tested more frequently, regardless of your age. If you have never gotten your cholesterol checked, and you're over the age of 20, make an appointment to do so as soon as possible, even if you don't have any of the risk factors mentioned above.

How Is a Cholesterol Test Done?

A cholesterol test can be done on a blood sample—not more than a pinprick—taken from your finger or arm. Your test results will come back in milligrams per deciliter (mg/dl) of blood.

For a complete lipid profile—which measures total cholesterol, HDL, LDL, and triglycerides (another type of blood fat)—you must fast for 9 to 12 hours before the blood sample is drawn. That means no food and no beverages except water, black coffee, or tea.

If your doctor thinks that any of the numbers in your test results are cause for concern, he will likely recommend a retest.

What Do the Test Results Mean?

The American Heart Association and *Prevention* offer the following guidelines for interpreting your cholesterol profile.

Total Cholesterol

Desirable: less than 200 mg/dl
Borderline high: 200 to 239 mg/dl
High: 240 mg/dl

If your total cholesterol is less than 200 mg/dl and you have no other risk factors, you're not very likely to develop heart disease. On the other hand, a reading in the borderline range is reason for caution. Even if you have no other risk factors, you should try to get your total cholesterol below 200 mg/dl.

If your total cholesterol falls in the high category, it's definitely a red flag. However, total cholesterol doesn't tell the whole story, since a high level of HDL (the good kind) can drive up your total cholesterol reading. If your total cholesterol comes back "high," be sure to find out exactly what levels of LDLs and HDLs you have, then talk with your doctor about whether you need to raise your HDLs, lower your LDLs, or both.

IT WORKED FOR ME!

Soy Helped Lower My Cholesterol 120 Points!

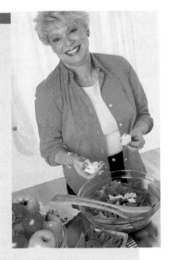

When Shelly Solomon cooks for her family, she doesn't reveal all the ingredients until the meal is over. That's because Shelly likes to sneak tofu into her meals. She puts it in chili, crumbles it into egg-substitute omelettes, and stashes it in casseroles. "You can stick tofu in anything, and it absorbs the flavor of whatever you're making," she says.

Shelly's cholesterol had hit a high of 280 in 1996. Even after taking the cholesterol-lowering drug Pravachol, giving up what little fat was left in her diet, and keeping up an exercise routine that included walking and yoga, her cholesterol was still 220. After eating soy every day for a year and continuing with Pravachol and her other good habits, today Shelly's cholesterol is a healthy 160.

These days, Shelly eats soy every other day—in the form of burgers, bacon, and chunks of tofu in her salads. And she continues to play food tricks on her family. "My boys think I'm nuts," she laughs. "They never know what I'm going to give them. I serve veggie chicken nuggets and Buffalo wings, and my family can't tell the difference! I take real pride in tricking them."

Research has proven that soy foods help lower cholesterol and reduce the risk of heart disease. In fact, the FDA allows food manufacturers of soy protein products to say so on their product labels.

LDL Cholesterol

Optimal: less than 100 mg/dl
Near optimal: 100 to 129 mg/dl
Borderline high: 130 to 159 mg/dl
High: 160 to 190 mg/dl
Very high: greater than 190 mg/dl

If your LDL cholesterol reading is in the borderline-high or high categories, your doctor will evaluate your other risk factors to determine if you need to lower your LDL level.

HDL Cholesterol

Desirable: 50 mg/dl or higher for women (40 mg/dl for men)

Your doctor will tell you if you need to raise your HDL level.

How Can I Lower My Cholesterol?

Most of the risk factors for high cholesterol are within your control. "Between diet and exercise, the average drop in cholesterol is 20 to 30%, but up to a 50% reduction is not unheard of," says Michael Miller, MD, associate professor of medicine and director of preventive cardiology at the University of Maryland School of Medicine in Baltimore. Here's how to make healthy choices.

Eat Less Saturated Fat

Once in your bloodstream, saturated fat prevents LDL cholesterol from properly breaking down in the liver, which drives your LDL level even higher. Even low-cholesterol or cholesterol-free foods may be bad for you if they contain a lot of saturated fat. You can make a big difference in your cholesterol levels and your heart disease risk

just by modifying your eating habits in the following ways.

Avoid
▶ meat
▶ full-fat dairy products
▶ oils high in saturated fat, such as coconut oil, palm kernel oil, and palm oil, all of which are common in processed foods. (Look at ingredients lists to see if these are present.)

Choose
▶ low-fat, high-fiber foods such as fruits, vegetables, and whole grains
▶ fish (which is full of heart-healthy omega-3 fatty acids)
▶ fat-free dairy products
▶ beans and soy products, such as tofu, soy milk, and meat alternatives.

Exercise Regularly

If you have high cholesterol, get moving! Among its many benefits, regular exercise can lower your LDL level, raise your HDL level, and help you maintain a healthy weight. Physical activity can also counter other risk factors for heart disease, including high blood pressure. See Part 2 of this book for some fast and effective workouts that offer great results for both your cholesterol level and your figure!

Don't Smoke

Smokers are more than twice as likely to have a heart attack as nonsmokers are. That's because cigarette smoke oxidizes LDL, making it more likely to form artery-clogging plaque. Even if you've been a longtime smoker, quitting for 2 years will drop your risk of heart attack to the level of someone who never smoked! If

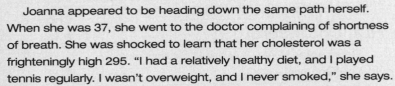

IT WORKED FOR ME!

Relaxation Lowered My Cholesterol 81 Points!

Speech communication professor Joanna Pucel routinely teaches others how to relax before presentations. But it took a cholesterol reading of 290 to convince her to put the brakes on her fast-paced lifestyle.

Stress wasn't the only factor putting Joanna at high risk for high cholesterol and heart disease. "My family history is horrendous," says the 54-year-old St. Cloud, MN, resident. "My mother's side of the family had 12 siblings, and most of my aunts and uncles died from heart attacks before they turned 30."

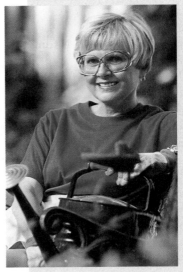

Joanna appeared to be heading down the same path herself. When she was 37, she went to the doctor complaining of shortness of breath. She was shocked to learn that her cholesterol was a frighteningly high 295. "I had a relatively healthy diet, and I played tennis regularly. I wasn't overweight, and I never smoked," she says.

Even though she seemed to be doing everything right, her arteries suggested otherwise. During an angiogram, her doctors detected a blocked coronary artery. They concluded that she was probably about a week away from a heart attack. In surgery, they made a more disturbing discovery: Joanna had suffered a silent heart attack years earlier, and part of her heart was no longer functioning.

She was determined to rein in her cholesterol. She switched from cooking oils to sprays and ate more fruit and bran. She invested in a treadmill that she used on the days that she didn't play tennis. Three years after surgery, with help from cholesterol-lowering drugs, her cholesterol finally dipped below 200.

Unfortunately, it didn't stay there. When she went through surgical menopause and lost the protective effects of estrogen, Joanna's cholesterol shot back up to 290. And none of her healthy habits were helping. "I kept asking myself, 'Why can't I get it down?' I felt I was missing something."

Through her own research, she uncovered a suspected connection between stress and cholesterol. She thought she'd found her culprit.

To cut down on stress, Joanna started setting priorities and cutting down on unnecessary obligations. She now makes time to go out to lunch with her tennis buddies and has taken up basket making. Every weekend, Joanna spends at least an hour puttering around in her greenhouse. And every night, she sets aside at least 15 minutes to soak in a steamy tub of water scented with her favorite bubble bath.

Judging by her latest cholesterol test, Joanna's stress-reduction efforts have been a success. Her total cholesterol is down to 209 with an LDL of 107 and an HDL of 91—a great ratio.

you need help kicking the habit, ask your doctor to help you find a plan or program that's right for you.

Maintain a Healthy Weight

The higher your body fat, the higher your LDL cholesterol. Excess pounds not only strain your heart, but they also affect your blood pressure and increase your odds of developing diabetes. Fortunately, eating healthier and exercising regularly—two habits that help lower cholesterol themselves—will also help you to lose excess pounds.

Lower Your Stress Level

Stress often leads to unhealthy habits such as overeating and smoking—two other recognized risk factors for high cholesterol. See "It Worked for Me: Relaxation Lowered My Cholesterol 81 Points!" at left for one woman's de-stressing success story.

Control High Blood Pressure and Diabetes

Both of these conditions raise your risk of heart disease. If you have either one, you should be under professional care. Your doctor can monitor your health status and adjust your treatment as necessary.

Consider Medications or Supplements

If the above measures fail to bring down your cholesterol levels, talk to your doctor about prescription medications such as statins and supplements such as saponins. Statins (such as lovastatin, pravastatin, and simvastatin) lower cholesterol by preventing your body from making a cholesterol-producing enzyme. Saponins, which are naturally found in some plants, latch onto cholesterol in the intestinal tract. Since your body can't absorb the saponins, they take the cholesterol out of your body as they exit. See "Do Just One Thing!" below for more on saponins.

DO JUST ONE THING!

Check Out This Natural Cholesterol Fighter

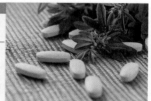

Cholesterol-lowering compounds called saponins are naturally found in several plants, but are especially rich in alfalfa, soybeans, chickpeas, and the yucca plant. Saponins are also found in herbs such as garlic, fenugreek, ginseng, red clover, and guaraná.

Your body can't absorb saponins, so when they latch onto cholesterol in the intestinal tract, they take the artery-clogging fat with them when they exit.

The research: Unpublished European studies show significant reductions in all the cholesterol-clogging fats and increases in the good HDLs. Another study found that monkeys taking alfalfa saponins experienced a reversal of the artery-clogging process and a healthy 50% drop in blood cholesterol levels.

How much to take: Follow package directions, and take saponins before you eat, especially if you're having high-fat foods. Don't take saponin supplements instead of prescription drugs. You'll get the most benefit if you take them together, but check with your doctor before taking any dietary supplement.

CHAPTER 13

Cut Your Cancer Risk As Much As 90%

Check out your current risks for common cancers— then learn how to slash them today!

Have you often had sunburns that blistered? You could be at risk for skin cancer. Do you have inflammatory bowel disease (IBS)? Colorectal cancer may be a risk for you. Does breast cancer run in your family? This may mean you should be extra vigilant with your own breast health. But none of these risk factors means that you *have* to wind up with cancer sometime in the future. In fact, decades of studies have shown that there are plenty of simple ways to lower your cancer risk *today*, and more recent studies are also revealing additional ways that even high-risk folks can lower their odds. Here's how to tell if you're at risk for breast, skin, and colorectal cancer—and how to bring that risk down.

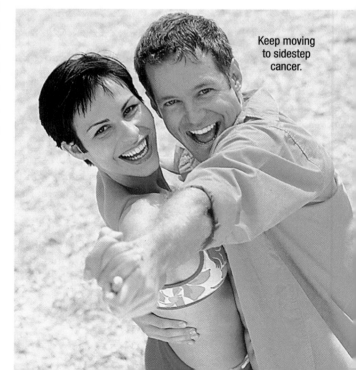

Keep moving to sidestep cancer.

‖ Breast Cancer

Having a close relative with breast cancer doubles a woman's risk of the disease, and having mutations in the genes known as BRCA1 and BRCA2 can boost it five-fold. "But just having the mutations doesn't necessarily mean you'll develop the disease," says Mary Fraser, a clinical nurse specialist and expert on heredity and cancer risk at the NCI. The way you live—what you eat, for instance—still seems to influence the odds. Here's how to lower your risk of getting or dying of breast cancer.

Keep Your Weight in Check
Reduce Your Risk 19%

If you avoid piling on the pounds, especially after menopause, according to the Nurses' Health Study, you can cut your risk 19%. Fat cells produce a form of estrogen that's been linked to an increased breast cancer risk, particularly after menopause, explains Michael Thun, MD, head of epidemiological research for the American Cancer Society.

Eat More Produce and Whole Grains
Reduce Your Risk 50%

According to an analysis of more than 200 studies, women who eat the most produce may cut their breast cancer risk in half. Shoot for nine servings of fruits and vegetables, and be sure to include the following.

Cruciferous vegetables, such as broccoli and cabbage, which are particularly rich in a cancer- fighting compound called sulforaphane.

Carrots, sweet potatoes, spinach, and other produce high in beta-carotene, a precursor of vitamin A. (These

1-MINUTE *HEALTH BOOSTER*

Limit Alcohol to Protect Your Breasts

Though alcohol may be good for your heart, having two or more drinks a day may boost your breast cancer risk by 41%, according to one study comparing drinkers with nondrinkers. Since there are better ways to protect your heart, limit yourself to two or three drinks a week.

foods are known for their antitumor effects, says Christine Pratt, PhD, a breast cancer expert and associate professor at the University of Ottawa.)

Also have 6 to 11 daily servings of whole grains. The insoluble fiber they provide helps rid your body of cancer-causing agents that boost breast cancer risk.

Get Regular Breast Exams
Reduce Your Risk 20 to 30%

Be sure to do the following, so you can catch cancer early if it does occur.

- ▶ Give yourself a monthly breast self-exam.
- ▶ Get a clinical breast exam every year once you turn 20.
- ▶ Schedule a baseline mammogram before age 40.
- ▶ Get a yearly mammogram after 40.

If You're High Risk

Here are factors that increase your risk.

- ▶ A close relative (particularly your mother, sister, or daughter) has been diagnosed with the disease.

Cut His Prostate Cancer Risk

Prostate cancer is the second most common cancer in American men. While there's still a lot that we don't know about treating or preventing it, some research suggests that men may be able to cut their risk of getting or dying from prostate cancer with the following lifestyle changes. Read on, then discuss them with the man in your life.

Increase the tomato products in his diet to cut risk 45%. Tomato products are rich in a cancer-fighting antioxidant called lycopene, which may lower prostate cancer risk. One preliminary study found that men with a weekly intake of 10 or more concentrated tomato products (such as tomato sauce and paste) had a 45% lower risk.

This pie's topped with cancer-fighting tomato sauce

Serve him soy to cut risk 35%. Japanese men, who eat far more soy than do US men, run a 35% lower risk of prostate cancer. Again, some experts say soy's benefits haven't been clearly established, but one person who recommends it is Mitchell Gaynor, MD, medical director at the Weill Cornell Center for Complementary and Integrative Medicine and author of *Dr. Gaynor's Cancer Prevention Program* (Kensington, 2000).

Add omega-3 fats to his diet to cut risk 40%. Serve your man at least one or two servings weekly of cold-water fish such as salmon, white albacore tuna, mackerel, and halibut, recommends Dr. Gaynor. (It's good for both of your hearts and waistlines too!)

Have him supplement his selenium intake to lower risk 65%. In one study of men living in areas with little of this nutrient in the soil, a 200-mcg supplement reduced the incidence of prostate cancer by about 65%.

Investigate vitamin E to cut risk over 30%. Some research suggests that 50 mg of vitamin E may lower your risk by about one-third.

Ask him about his family history. The man in your life may run an increased risk of prostate cancer if a close relative (a brother or his father) has prostate cancer or if he has been diagnosed with mutations in BRCA1 and 2 genes. Other risk factors include being older (more than 70% of cases are diagnosed after age 65) or being African-American. If your man has a family history of prostate cancer or other risk factors, along with the above risk reduction advice, he should also get screened yearly.

Talk to him about getting checked. It's a good idea for men to talk to their doctor about the benefits and liabilities of having a digital rectal exam (DRE) and a prostate-specific antigen (PSA) screening test. Routine screening is controversial, since studies have yet to show that screening programs prevent deaths from prostate cancer, although preliminary studies suggest they can. *Prevention* recommends an annual DRE and PSA for Caucasian men starting at age 50 and for African-Americans starting at 40.

▶ You've been diagnosed with certain non-cancerous breast abnormalities.

▶ You got your period before age 11.

▶ You went through menopause after the age of 55.

▶ You're postmenopausal and obese.

▶ You've used oral contraceptives or hormone replacement therapy for more than 10 years.

▶ You've never had children or had your first child after turning 35.

If you have a family history of breast cancer or any of the other risk factors listed above, see "Improve Your Odds" on p. 88. There, you'll learn about the benefits of receiving genetic counseling, getting annual mammograms starting at age 35 or younger, and learning about drugs and surgeries that can help reduce your risk.

‖ Skin Cancer

The most common cancer in the US would be far less common if everyone took some basic precautions, says Homer Black, PhD, a professor of dermatology at Baylor College of Medicine in Houston. You may be able to cut your risk of getting or dying of skin cancer by following these precautions.

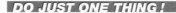
DO JUST ONE THING!

Give Your Skin the Once-Over

When checking for new moles and skin growths or changes in old ones, look for these "ABCD" warning signs:

Asymmetry: One-half of the growth doesn't mirror the other half.

Border irregularity: The growth has ragged or blurry edges.

Color variations: A mole that, for example, is tan in one area and brown in another.

Diameters: Growths bigger than a pencil eraser or growing.

Avoid Excessive Sun Exposure
Reduce Your Risk 90%

By limiting your time in the sun, you can cut your risk for skin cancer dramatically. Here's what to do.

▶ Stay out of the sun, particularly between 10 AM and 4 PM, when it's most intense. Don't make exceptions. Brief periods of high sun exposure, such as a weeklong vacation in Barbados, seem to *increase* the risk of a potentially deadly type of skin cancer called melanoma.

▶ Avoid tanning beds for the same reason.

▶ When outdoors during daylight hours, wear a hat, sunglasses, sunscreen with an SPF of at least 15, and when possible, a long-sleeved shirt and pants.

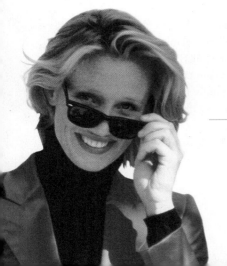

Stay in the shade between 10 AM and 4 PM, and cut your skin cancer risk 90%!

Cut Your Fat Intake
Reduce Your Risk 75%

In a 2-year study tracking 115 people previously treated for skin cancer, Dr. Black and colleagues found that those who cut fat consumption from 36% to 20% of calories cut their risk of precancerous skin growths by 75%. Bonus: This habit is also good for your heart, your waistline, and every other part of your body!

Examine Your Skin
Reduce Your Risk 34%

Every couple of months, check your skin for new moles or other growths and changes in existing ones, suggests Boris Bastian, MD, assistant professor at the University of California at San Francisco's Comprehensive Cancer Center. (See "Give Your Skin the Once-Over" on p. 99.) The study that established

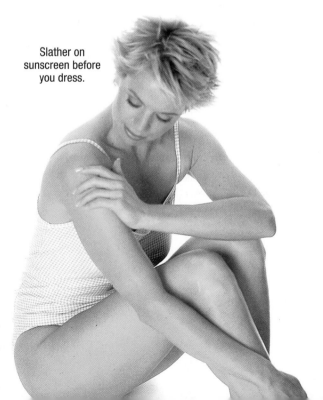

Slather on sunscreen before you dress.

What Do the Numbers Mean?

The percentages we used to measure the reduced risk of the cancers discussed in this chapter are drawn from the results of scientific studies, often, but not always, of large groups of people. There's no guarantee that you can reduce your own odds by these percentages, but the recommendations of cancer experts interviewed for this article have all been shown to be helpful in lowering cancer risk.

this percentage referred to malignant melanoma, the most serious of the skin cancers. Suspicious growths can be precancerous or cancerous, and the earlier they're treated, the better. Also be sure to

▶ have a dermatologist check anything suspicious.

▶ see a dermatologist for a check every 3 years before 40, and every year after that.

If You're High Risk

Here are factors that increase your skin cancer risk:

▶ Your family tree has roots in the United Kingdom or Ireland.

▶ Irregularly shaped moles run in your family.

▶ You have fair skin or freckles.

▶ You've had blistering sunburns, lots of moles, or irregularly shaped moles.

▶ You've had skin cancer previously.

If you have a family history of skin cancer or any of the other risk factors listed here, you should also do skin self-exams once a month, and see a dermatologist at least once a year, regardless of your age.

‖ Colon Cancer

Every year, more than 135,000 Americans are diagnosed with colon cancer, and more than 48,000 die of the disease. About half of those deaths could be prevented, the experts estimate, if we all followed some basic advice.

Exercise Regularly

Reduce Your Risk 50%

According to the Atlanta-based American Cancer Society, all it takes to halve your risk is getting at least 30 minutes of activity most days. See Chapter 8 for a great walking program to help you do just that.

Trim Down to Your Ideal Weight

Reduce Your Risk 40%

Eating healthfully and exercising regularly can help you trim down to your ideal weight—and thereby reduce your colorectal cancer risk by a considerable amount. Talk with your doctor if you're not sure what your ideal weight is.

Modify Your Diet

Reduce Your Risk 34%

People who eat lots of fruits and vegetables but little fatty meat and rarely, if ever, drink appear to run a lower risk of colon cancer. Here's what to shoot for:

- ▶ Eat 5 (preferably 9) servings of fruits and vegetables daily.
- ▶ Limit your red-meat consumption to just one serving each week.
- ▶ Have no more than one alcoholic drink per day. (And the man in your life should have no more than 2 drinks daily.)

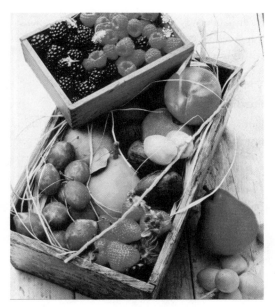

These antioxidant-rich nuggets are Mother Nature's anti-cancer medicine!

Take Nutritional Supplements

Reduce Your Risk 75%

Adding the following dietary supplements to your daily regimen may help keep colon cancer at bay:

- ▶ A daily multivitamin that packs 400 micrograms (mcg) of folic acid
- ▶ An additional supplement of 1,200 mg of calcium per day

The data on the benefits of a daily multi comes from the Nurses' Health Study, an ongoing study tracking nearly 60,000 nurses. Also, another large study showed that people taking a 1,200-mg calcium supplement daily had a 20% lower risk of precancerous adenomas. More studies are underway to determine if this effect can be improved by combining calcium with other cancer-fighting agents.

Get Regular Screenings
Reduce Your Risk 50%

Get a digital rectal exam and fecal occult blood test every year after 50 and a colonoscopy every 10 years, or a sigmoidoscopy every 3 to 5 years.

If You're High Risk

Here are factors that increase your colorectal cancer risk:

▶ The disease or precancerous polyps run in your family.

▶ You've been diagnosed with polyps.

▶ You have inflammatory bowel disease.

▶ You've been diagnosed with genetic mutations associated with two types of the disease: familial adenomatous polyposis (FAP) or hereditary nonpolyposis colon cancer (HNPCC).

If you have a family history of colon cancer or any of the other risk factors mentioned above, see "Improve Your Odds" on p. 88 for additional measures to help you stay cancer-free. They include earlier and more frequent screenings, genetic counseling and testing, and a medication called celecoxib that may help prevent the development of precancerous colorectal polyps.

CHAPTER 14

Stop Diabetes Before It Starts

Is a silent killer at work in your body?
Here's how to tell—and what to do

Three years ago, Maureen Marinelli learned that she had a disease she didn't even know was a disease. She was diagnosed with impaired glucose tolerance, a symptom-less condition in which blood sugar rises higher than normal—enough to put you at risk of serious complications but not quite high enough to fit current definitions of type 2 diabetes.

Maureen is far from alone. In fact, 20 to 30 million Americans probably have impaired glucose tolerance, and most of them don't know they have it. In fact, *you* could be among them. And those who *do* know they have it often dismiss it as "a touch of sugar" or "borderline diabetes." Their doctors may call it "impaired fasting glucose" or "impaired glucose tolerance" (depending on what test

Diabetes
can strike
at any age.

was used to diagnose it)—but often they don't treat it aggressively. And that's unfortunate, because this condition, which *Prevention* calls "early diabetes," can lead to full-blown diabetes, a life-threatening disease that can lead to heart attack, stroke, kidney failure, circulatory problems, blindness, amputation, even bone fractures and depression.

For Maureen, diabetes and all of its complications are less of a risk now, because she has made some simple lifestyle changes that have lowered her blood sugar and, in turn, her risk for diabetes. With the information in this chapter, you, like Maureen, can have a healthier future too.

‖ What Is Diabetes?

An estimated 16 million Americans have diabetes, and at least one-third are undiagnosed and untreated. When you have diabetes, something is wrong with your production of insulin, a hormone produced by your pancreas. Insulin helps your cells take in fuel in the form of blood sugar. This blood sugar, also called glucose, is produced when your body digests food. If glucose doesn't get into the cells, they begin to weaken. Then the sugar from your food builds up in your bloodstream, damaging everything from your blood vessels to your organs. A small percentage of people have type 1 diabetes, in which the body doesn't produce insulin, but most people with diabetes—90 to 95%—have type 2: Their body isn't able to use the insulin that's produced, and the pancreas may also produce less insulin over time.

‖ What Is *Early* Diabetes?

If your blood sugar is higher than normal but not in the range for full-blown diabetes, you have early diabetes. This condition

▶ raises your risk of full-blown, type 2 diabetes by 50% over 10 years

- potentially doubles your risk of heart disease
- triples your risk of high blood pressure
- makes you five times more likely to die from a heart attack
- may be linked to some forms of cancer

But these dangers are often downplayed—if they're mentioned at all. "I call it the Rodney Dangerfield of human diseases. It doesn't get any respect," says John Buse, MD, PhD, CDE (Certified Diabetes Educator), associate professor of medicine at the University of North Carolina School of Medicine in Chapel Hill, and director of the university's Diabetes Care Center.

Risk Factors for Early Diabetes

Genetics may account for 15 to 20% of diabetes and early diabetes risk. There's even new evidence that chronic lack of sleep can make you susceptible. But the real culprit is our high-fat, high-stress, no-time-for-exercise way of life and the epidemic of obesity that's come with it. Studies show that obesity raises diabetes risk by up to 93%. And inactivity alone raises the risk by 25%.

The Fat Connection

Fifty-five percent of Americans are overweight, and more than one-quarter are obese. More kids are overweight too. As a result, diabetes is on the rise and is becoming more common among younger people as well. The Centers for Disease Control and Prevention estimates that the number of people in their 30s with type 2 diabetes has increased 70%. Among children, the disease has increased tenfold in the past 5 years.

1-MINUTE *HEALTH BOOSTER*

Assess Your Diabetes Risk

You're at risk for diabetes if you

- are overweight, or have a body mass index (BMI) of 25 or more.*
- carry fat around your waist and belly
- exercise infrequently or not at all
- are age 45 or older (being over 65 raises your risk even higher)
- have a family history of type 2 diabetes
- had diabetes when you were pregnant
- had a baby weighing 9 lb or more
- are African-American, Latino, Asian-American, or Native American
- have high triglycerides (greater than 250)
- have high blood pressure (140/90 or above)

*To estimate your BMI: Multiply your weight (in pounds) by 703. Multiply your height (in inches) by itself. Divide your first answer by your second answer.

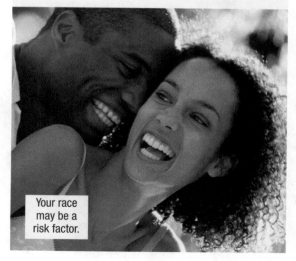

Your race may be a risk factor.

The Stress Connection

When you're under stress, your body produces high levels of a stress hormone called cortisol. This hormone causes your body to store fat around your middle, packed around your internal organs. Research suggests that this belly fat—known as visceral fat—may be an even more potent risk factor for diabetes than weight alone.

A study of 678 African-American and Hispanic people with a family history of diabetes found that regardless of age, gender, or weight, visceral fat was the most powerful factor determining who had insulin resistance—the body's lack of sensitivity to insulin that causes early diabetes.

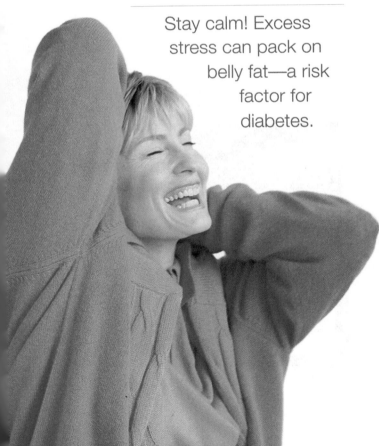

Stay calm! Excess stress can pack on belly fat—a risk factor for diabetes.

The Combination Effect

"Overweight, a high-fat diet, and visceral fat all intertwine to produce insulin resistance," says Dr. Buse. "We don't completely understand the process yet, but one theory is that people who are insulin resistant are storing excess dietary fat in all kinds of inappropriate places, such as in muscle cells and in the liver, which makes it harder for their body to use sugar as fuel," he adds.

Scientists suspect that during early diabetes, high insulin levels may raise heart disease risk into the danger zone by thickening artery walls and raising blood pressure. And insulin resistance is linked to the development of a very lethal kind of bad cholesterol—small, dense LDLs—that sets the stage for heart disease.

The Test You Need to Have—Now

Early diabetes is easy to detect with a simple blood check called a *fasting plasma glucose test*. After an 8- to 12-hour fast, your blood is drawn, and blood sugar level measured. A reading of 109 mg/dl or less is normal; 110 to 125 is called impaired fasting glucose; 126 or higher is a sign of full-blown diabetes.

Another check, called an *oral glucose tolerance test,* involves drinking a sugared beverage and getting a blood sugar check after 2 hours. If your reading is between 140 and 199 mg/dl, you have impaired glucose tolerance; 200 or higher indicates diabetes.

Which test is better? New evidence suggests that the oral glucose tolerance test may catch early diabetes sooner—and may also be a more accurate test for people over age 65.

Who should be tested? Probably everyone.

Prevention's "Fight Diabetes Before It Starts" Plan

Don't wait! Diabetes experts say these easy steps can dramatically reduce your risk of diabetes or reverse early diabetes.

Get tested now. See the risk factors and testing information on pp. 105 and 106.

Get retested in 6 months to a year to find out if your risk has gone up or down.

Nudge the scale. In a Finnish study, even extremely overweight people lowered their risk of diabetes by 70% when they lost just 5% of their total weight—even if they didn't exercise. If you weigh 175 lb, that's a little less than 9 lb. See Parts 1 and 2 of this book for weight loss tips that work.

Cut the fat. Targets for healthy fat intake range from less than 30% of daily calories (less than 10% saturated fat) to a daily 42 g fat. *Prevention* recommends keeping total fat intake to 25% of your daily calories.

Eat more fruits, veggies, and whole grains. *Prevention* recommends nine servings of fruits and vegetables a day. Try to chose whole grains for at least half of your starches (including breads, rice, and pasta) to raise your fiber intake still higher.

Move a little more. People in the Finnish study who exercised the most—up to 4 hours a week—dropped their risk of diabetes by 80%, even if they didn't lose any weight. America's Diabetes Prevention Program (DPP) aimed for just 30 minutes of exercise, five times a week, and got big results. Moderate exercise—walking, biking, playing tennis—is enough to improve your odds.

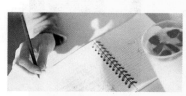

Keep a food diary. In both studies, keeping a food diary kept participants on track toward eating better. List what you eat, the portion sizes, and the fat grams.

Enlist a coach. The secret to the success of study volunteers in both research projects was regular interaction with a registered dietitian/lifestyle counselor. "She became like my shrink, helping me get through stressful times without overeating and figuring out how to help me get past obstacles to healthier habits," says DPP participant Maureen Marinelli.

Your insurance plan may not cover nutrition counseling if you're diagnosed with early diabetes. But it may if you have another health problem such as high cholesterol, high triglycerides, high blood pressure, or obesity. It's worth asking. Otherwise, try a program such as Weight Watchers, which offers nutrition counseling as part of its membership benefits.

But if you fit the high-risk profile for diabetes (see "Assess Your Diabetes Risk" on p. 105), you should get tested as soon as possible. Your family doctor can schedule both types of tests.

Stack the Deck in Your Favor

You can lower your risk of getting full-blown diabetes 80 to 100% by losing as little as 5% of your body weight—as little as 8 lb if you weigh 160, for example, and exercising as little as half an hour a day. As a bonus, you'll also slash your heart disease risk.

That's what happened in the Finnish Diabetes Prevention Study, when 523 extremely overweight people with impaired glucose tolerance tried an easy-does it, five-point plan.

▶ Get half an hour of exercise daily.
▶ Lose 5% of your total weight.
▶ Reduce your fat intake to 30% of total calories.

DO JUST ONE THING!

Modify Workouts to Stabilize Blood Sugar

For people with diabetes, exercise is medicine. "Blood glucose levels can drop 20 to 30% after a single exercise session," says Cathy Mullooly, director of exercise physiology at Joslin Diabetes Center in Boston. It's a good idea to check with your doctor before beginning any exercise regimen, especially if you haven't worked out before. Here's how to customize your workout if you have diabetes or early diabetes.

▶ **Walk regularly.** If you're walking mainly to control blood sugar, move at a slow to moderate pace for 20 to 30 minutes, three or four times a week. To lose weight and lower your risk of other diseases, build up to walking at a moderate pace for 45 to 60 minutes at least five times a week. Tackle hills or do speed intervals if it's comfortable.

▶ **Modify your routine if you have complications.** If you have pain in your legs or feet or peripheral vascular disease, walk 10 minutes at a time, three or four times a day. Or try a non–weight bearing activity such as water walking in a pool.

▶ **Eat something 30 minutes before exercising.**

▶ **Don't allow more than a 48-hour lapse between sessions.**

▶ **Walk at the same time each day.**

▶ **And if you have full-blown diabetes, check your blood sugar levels before and after walking to help prevent dangerous dips.**

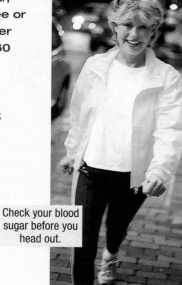

Check your blood sugar before you head out.

▶ Cut your saturated fat intake to less than 10% of total calories.

▶ Eat more fiber (more fruits, veggies, and whole grains).

Those who took four of the five steps didn't develop diabetes at all. Those who lost the weight and reached two other goals reduced their risk by more than 70%. And those who said they exercised consistently and succeeded at reaching at least two other goals cut their risk by 80%.

"Of course we celebrated when we got the results," says lead investigator Jaakko Tuomilehto, MD, PhD, academy professor in the diabetes and genetic epidemiology unit of Finland's National Public Health Institute in Helsinki. "We think the biggest, long-range health benefits will probably be the reduction in the risk of cardiovascular and renal [kidney] complications and reduction in the risk of all other major diabetes complications."

Americans should expect the same results, say US researchers, who recently released the findings of the landmark $174 million Diabetes Prevention Program (DPP) a study that was ended a year early because the results were so dramatic. Among its 3,224 participants (all of whom had impaired glucose tolerance), those who lost 5 to 7% of their body weight and exercised for half an hour a day reduced their risk of developing full-blown, type 2 diabetes by a whopping 58%. In contrast, those who took a diabetes drug improved their odds by only 31%.

"Every year that a person can live free of dia-

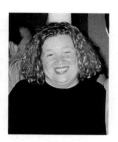

Maureen Marinelli used dancing and diet to slash her risk!

betes means an added year of life free of suffering, disability, and the medical costs incurred by this disease," says Edward Horton, MD, professor of medicine at Harvard Medical School and director of clinical research at the Joslin Diabetes Center in Boston, where he is lead investigator for Joslin's part in the DPP.

She Did It— So Can You!

Maureen Marinelli volunteered for the DPP study, because "I didn't want to cross that line into diabetes."

With the help of a nutrition and lifestyle counselor, she lost 18 lb. She now eats more fruits, veggies, and whole grains. She tap-dances two or three times a week. As a result, she expects to keep her risk of diabetes and heart disease in the "normal" range for life.

"I feel good about what I'm doing," she says. "I have more energy. And I'm protecting my health."

CHAPTER 15

Beat Rheumatoid Arthritis!

Breakthrough treatments can ease the joint pain that targets young women

Think you're too young to get arthritis? Think again. A common form of joint inflammation known as rheumatoid arthritis (RA) is an autoimmune disorder that affects more than 2 million Americans, mostly women between the ages of 20 and 45. Symptoms also include joint pain, stiffness, fatigue, and even feverishness.

In the past decade, there's been an explosion in the understanding and treatment of RA—the most important discovery being that early diagnosis, followed by early aggressive treatment, will help people with RA live longer, healthier lives with less pain, less joint damage, and less likelihood of permanent disability. That's why it's important that women who *don't* have RA become familiar with its symptoms—so they can seek treatment early if they do develop it.

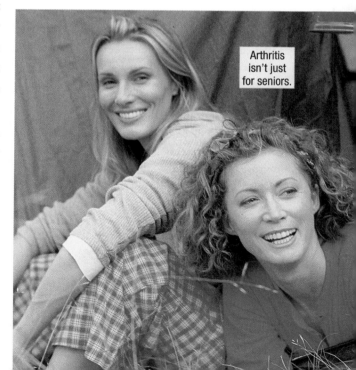

Arthritis isn't just for seniors.

For reasons that aren't clear, the body's immune system turns against itself and attacks healthy joint tissue. The resulting inflammation can lead to irreversible destruction of bone and cartilage. And it can be disabling: About half of the people with RA are unable to work within 10 years of onset.

Genes play a key role in determining who gets RA and who doesn't. Genes most likely also explain why some people have more severe disease than others. But genes don't provide all the answers. One theory is that environmental factors, such as a virus or bacteria, "turn on" RA in people with an inherited susceptibility.

Even if you've had RA for years, you can benefit from the new medications available for

DO JUST ONE THING!

Learn the Symptoms

Diagnosing RA can be challenging. Many of RA's hallmark signs and symptoms such as fatigue and joint pain are shared by other health conditions, including other forms of arthritis. Also symptoms may come and go early on, making diagnosis difficult.

RA typically involves the same joints on both sides of the body. The hands, wrists, feet, knees, ankles, shoulders, neck, jaw, and elbows may be affected. Rheumatologists typically use the following guidelines to evaluate patients for RA, which may be diagnosed if at least four of the following criteria are met.

- ▶ Morning stiffness in and around the joints lasting at least 1 hour before maximum improvement.
- ▶ At least three joint areas with simultaneous soft tissue swelling or fluid.
- ▶ At least one joint area swollen, as defined above, in a wrist, knuckle, or the middle joint of a finger.
- ▶ Simultaneous involvement of the same joint areas on both sides of the body.
- ▶ Rheumatoid nodules (lumps of tissue) under the skin.
- ▶ Rheumatoid factor in the blood. (Approximately 80% of people with RA test positive for the presence of rheumatoid factor, an antibody found in the blood. However, the absence or presence of rheumatoid factor does not indicate that one has RA.)
- ▶ X-ray evidence of erosions (wearing away of the surface of bone) is typical of rheumatoid arthritis in the hand or wrist joints.
- ▶ Other possible symptoms include loss of appetite, fever, loss of energy, and anemia.

Sources: American College of Rheumatology and Arthritis Foundation

treating RA. You may even be able to do things that you never dreamed possible!

If you suspect you may have RA, turn to "Learn the Symptoms" on p. 111. If you *know* you've got it, read on for the breakthrough medications that can bring relief.

Important Shifts in Treatment

In past years, it was standard for doctors to hold off prescribing more powerful drugs for as long as possible to spare patients some of the more potent side effects, which can include liver damage, kidney damage, and blood problems.

Now doctors know that RA can cause permanent disability within a few years or even months, so they're quickly putting patients on what are called disease-modifying, anti-rheumatic drugs (DMARD), a more aggressive therapy that's now the gold standard in RA patient care.

When you have RA, chances are you'll be taking at least two different kinds of drugs:

▶ Those that reduce your symptoms—such as corticosteroids or nonsteroidal anti-inflammatories (NSAIDs)

▶ Those that slow progression of the disease before your joints are damaged (the DMARDs)

While NSAIDs and steroids provide fast relief, DMARDs work over time, sometimes taking several weeks to several months before patients and their doctors know if they're going to help. They're often used in combination with other RA drugs.

Among the most commonly prescribed are methotrexate (Rheumatrex), sulfasalazine (Azulfidine), and hydroxychloroquine (Plaquenil). Leflunomide (Arava) is one of the newest DMARDs. Approved in 1999, Arava inhibits the immune system, which is involved in the inflammatory process. (Several other drugs, including methotrexate, also target the immune system.)

DMARDs have been lifesavers for many people with RA, bringing relief from symptoms and slowing down the disease. But they often have intolerable side effects, and not one has produced what rheumatologists and their patients have been searching for: long-term remission.

New Drugs, Fewer Side Effects

The newest DMARDs may solve some of these problems. They're so different that they have their own classification: biologic response modifiers (BRM). Since 1998, the first three BRMs, commonly called "biologics," have been introduced: etanercept (Enbrel), infliximab (Remicade), and anakinra (Kineret).

These so-called biologics interrupt the inflammation process by blocking the action of certain proteins associated with swelling and joint damage in people with RA. Unlike most other

Natural Therapies That Really Work!

Complementary therapies won't make it possible for you to throw away your drugs. But many can help patients live better lives, says James McKoy, MD, chief of rheumatology and director of the integrative medicine service at Kaiser Permanente in Honolulu. If you decide to use a complementary therapy, make sure you discuss it with your doctor. Certain therapies may have an adverse reaction with medications. Also some therapies may be covered by your health insurance plan with your doctor's referral.

Mind/body medicine. A variety of stress-relieving techniques can help with chronic pain management, including meditation, biofeedback, breathing exercises, and massage therapy.

Exercise. People with RA can exercise when their joints are not inflamed. Regular exercise increases flexibility and strength, fights fatigue, and improves bone density, which is important because RA itself is a risk factor for osteoporosis, as is the use of corticosteroids for RA. Consider both traditional exercises such as walking and water aerobics and alternative forms of exercise such as yoga and tai chi.

Water workouts are easier on joints.

Nutrition and diet. Start with a high-potency multivitamin, and fill your plate with whole, unprocessed foods, such as whole grains, legumes, vegetables, fruits, nuts, and seeds. Also be sure to cut back on saturated animal fats and polyunsaturated vegetable oils such as corn and soybean oils, which can increase inflammation, and use more good fats, including olive oil, omega-3 essential fatty acids from fish, and flaxseed oil. In numerous studies, omega-3 fatty acids from fish and flaxseed oil have been shown to reduce the pain and stiffness of RA. You may need to get about 6 g of omega-3s a day. Consider taking a fish-oil capsule, but check with your doctor first if you are on blood-thinning medication.

Green tea. Both regular and decaffeinated green tea contains polyphenols, which have anti-inflammatory properties. Three to four cups a day are safe.

Herbal remedies. Dr. McKoy will sometimes prescribe turmeric and ginger, two anti-inflammatory herbs. However, there are few good studies that show a statistically significant benefit.

Biologics: The Newest RA Fighters

Here's a handy guide to the newest class of RA medications. They aren't pills—all must be taken by self-injection or an intravenous infusion (done by a doctor).

Etanercept (Enbrel)

What it does: Delays structural damage and reduces signs and symptoms of moderately to severely active RA

Who's getting it: People who haven't responded to other drugs; children with unresponsive juvenile RA; people whose insurance covers it; can also be used as a first line agent and experimentally for lupus, psoriatic arthritis, and other autoimmune diseases

Side effects: Local irritation at the site of injection; concerns that it curbs the inflammatory response, so it may make it harder to fight infection

Cost: About $225 per week for two 25-mg injections, or $10,000 to $12,000 a year

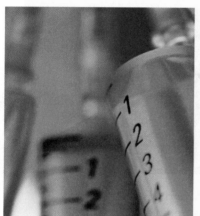

The newest RA drugs have fewer side effects to consider.

Infliximab (Remicade)

What it does: Delays structural damage and reduces signs and symptoms of moderately to severely active RA

Who's getting it: Used in combination with methotrexate in people with moderate to severe RA who haven't shown much improvement with methotrexate; people with Crohn's disease

Side effects: Same concerns about infection as etanercept

Cost: About $1,222 for each 8-week dose (dose is based on patient's body weight plus cost of infusion)

Anakinra (Kineret)

What it does: Reduces signs and symptoms of moderate to severe RA

Who's getting it: Used alone or in combination with a DMARD such as methotrexate in adult patients who have failed with one or more DMARDs, or other biologics

Side effects: Pain and swelling at injection site; same infection concerns as etanercept and infliximab

Cost: $11,088 for a year's supply of injections

RA drugs, the biologics aren't pills. They're proteins that must be taken either by self-injection, as diabetics take insulin, or by intravenous infusion, which must be done by a doctor.

But the biggest difference between biologics and other DMARDs is that biologics have fewer side effects. That's because, unlike their earlier cousins, they target only the parts of the immune system that contribute to RA.

The Pros and Cons of the New Drugs

At least two of the biologics, Enbrel and Remicade, either alone or in combination with methotrexate, appear to work faster and may produce better results than methotrexate alone.

"There's good evidence that biologic agents are superior to traditional DMARDs in preventing joint damage," says John Klippel, MD, medical director of the Atlanta-based Arthritis Foundation.

In one study done at Johns Hopkins University in Baltimore, for example, the biologic agent Enbrel stopped disease progression in 72% of the RA patients who injected it twice a week for a year, while just 60% had similar improvement taking methotrexate pills.

One downside to biologics is cost, which ranges from approximately $10,000 to $12,000 a year. Medicare pays for Remicade, which requires intravenous infusion at the doctor's office. But it doesn't cover Enbrel or Kineret, which are self-injected.

Questions also remain about the safety and long-term efficacy of biologics, because they're so new. The most common side effects appear to be susceptibility to infection, redness, and irritation and pain at the injection site. (See "Biologics: The Newest RA Fighters" at left.)

What Treatment Is Right for You?

Of course, with more options, the decision on which treatment is best for you is more challenging. How will you and your doctor decide? A lot will depend on the severity of your disease and how rapidly it progresses. Also to be factored in: how well you're doing with the drugs you're on, side effects, insurance coverage, and cost.

Though the new drugs are an exciting development, about two-thirds of people with RA are already helped dramatically by traditional drugs. But if you're in that remaining one-third who aren't helped by these treatments, the new drugs offer hope that you can stop RA from taking control of your life.

CHAPTER 16

Are Your Bones As Strong As You Think?

Four cutting-edge breakthroughs that you and your doctor should be aware of

Are your bones in good hands? Before you say yes, consider these facts:

▶ In a study of 1,162 postmenopausal women who sought medical care for a wrist fracture—a telltale sign of osteoporosis—only one-quarter were given further evaluation or treatment.

▶ Out of 502 women with a hip fracture—another telltale sign—almost none of them were given a bone-density test, according to another study.

▶ After their bone-density tests showed they had osteoporosis, 20% of the women in another study received no follow-up treatment.

▶ In a survey of 1,000 women with osteoporosis, 86% said they had never discussed osteoporosis prevention with their doctor.

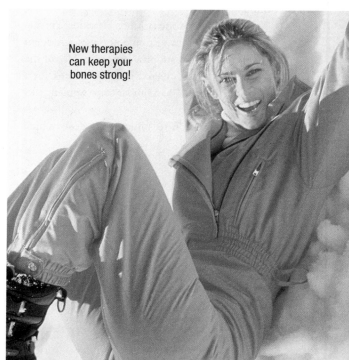

New therapies can keep your bones strong!

What's going on here? It's not wholesale apathy among doctors, it's just that many were never trained to catch the signs of osteoporosis or to treat it. And if your doctor is one of them, you could be in trouble.

Knowing about new, cutting-edge developments could help you prevent this debilitating disease or get the kind of treatment that can help you prevent its most serious consequences—a crippling hump, fractures, and even death. Check out the red flags on the pages that follow. If one of them sounds like your situation, make an appointment with your doctor—and take this book with you.

A heel or finger bone-density test says you're "normal."

What your doctor needs to know: You could still have osteoporosis. The readings you get on smaller peripheral bone-density devices that measure the heel, finger, wrist, or hand may not be as reliable as a hip measurement from a dual energy x-ray absorptiometry test (known as a central DEXA).

Here's why: When you get a central DEXA of the hip, your risk of fracture—and, ultimately, whether or not you are diagnosed with osteoporosis—is determined by comparing your results with the normal bone density of a healthy young adult of the same sex. The result, called a T-score, determines your risk. No matter what central DEXA machine you use, your hip results are compared with the same standard database of "healthy, young, normal," so the T-score for your hip should be the same on each machine.

But there are 20 different types of peripheral machines used, and each has a different "healthy,

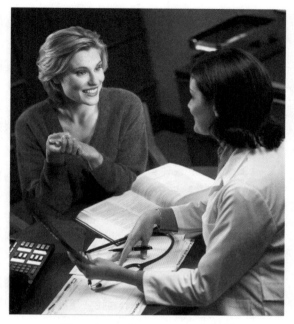

Fractured your ankle?
Ask for a bone-density
test right away!

young, normal" database. (DEXA spine measurements currently don't use a standardized database either.) So your score could vary depending on the machine you use. In fact, it's possible that you'd have a normal reading on one machine, another could put you at high risk, and yet another could diagnose you with osteoporosis, says Paul D. Miller, MD, medical director of the Colorado Center for Bone Research in Lakewood.

Bone density can also vary from place to place in your body. So a normal reading at your heel doesn't necessarily indicate that your hip is in good shape.

What to do: Obviously, such a false sense of security could be dangerous. That's why Dr. Miller and various experts are working on a universal database for all peripheral machines as well as a way to figure out what a T-score reading at a peripheral site translates to elsewhere in the body. Until these projects are completed (an estimated year or more from now), here's what to do with your test results.

▶ If you score -1 or lower, ask your doctor about further central DEXA testing.

▶ If you score between −1 and +1, ask for further testing if you have major risk factors for osteoporosis such as a history of fractures in your immediate family, if you smoke, if you weigh less than 127 lb, if you take steroid medication, or if you've had a previous fracture.

▶ If you score between −1 and +1 but you do not have major risk factors, you don't need further testing right now. Get another peripheral test in 1 year.

▶ If you score a +1 or higher, you're fine. You can wait a year or two before getting another peripheral test.

▶ If you're over 40, and you break a bone, ask your doctor for a central DEXA test and treatment options—no matter what reading a peripheral test gives you.

DO JUST ONE THING!

Get a Bone-Density Test

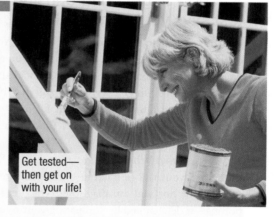

Get tested—
then get on
with your life!

Osteoporosis can sneak up on you, because you can't see or feel your bones weakening. But a bone-density test can catch osteoporosis before a debilitating hip or spinal fracture occurs, when preventive treatment will be most effective.

The best type of test is a central DEXA, which measures bone at both the hip and spine. Tell your doctor that you want to get tested if you meet any of these requirements:

▶ You're a woman age 65 or older.

▶ You're a postmenopausal woman and have one of these risk factors for osteoporosis: family history, smoke or drink excessive amounts of alcohol, don't get enough calcium, are inactive, are underweight, or have taken steroids or other medications that may thin your bones.

▶ You've had a fracture as an adult that wasn't caused by severe trauma.

Prevention recommends that women have a baseline bone-density test at the first signs of menopause—or earlier if you have one or more of the risk factors for osteoporosis listed above. If you're 50 or older, the test may be covered by your health insurance.

You're a premenopausal woman with low bone density, and your doctor has prescribed a bone-preserving drug.

What your doctor needs to know: You should not be taking a bone-preserving drug unless it's been determined that you are actually losing bone. Bisphosphonates such as Fosamax and Actonel prevent bone loss. So does a different type of drug, the calcitonin nasal spray Miacalcin. These are wonderful treatment options for post-menopausal women who may be losing bone as their estrogen levels dwindle.

But premenopausal women—even those with low bone density—are not necessarily *losing* bone, says Felicia Cosman, MD, clinical director at the National Osteoporosis Foundation in Washington, DC. You may have scored low because you never built much bone during your peak mass-building years, but that doesn't mean you're losing bone now. And if you're not losing bone, taking a bone-preserving drug won't help. In fact, there's no research on the safety or long-term effects of these drugs in premenopausal women.

What to do: If your doctor recommends a bone-preserving drug, and you are pre-menopausal, tell him no—unless he can prove through simple and standard urine and blood testing that you are indeed losing bone.

You're taking 10 mg Fosamax every morning, but the strict dosage directions are interfering with your routine.

What your doctor needs to know: You can now take a single 70-mg dose of Fosamax

1-MINUTE HEALTH BOOSTER

On the Pill? Take *Extra* Calcium!

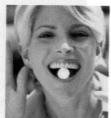

Calculate your ideal calcium intake.

If you're on birth control pills, exercise—which is known to keep bones strong—may not be enough for you, according to research from Purdue University in West Lafayette, IN.

In a 2-year study of 55 women, ages 18 to 30, researchers found that those who jumped rope and lifted weights 3 days a week increased their total bone density by 1 to 2%, while those who didn't exercise lost that much. But exercisers who took oral contraceptives and didn't get adequate calcium actually *lost* bone in their hips and spine—two important sites that can be at high risk for debilitating fractures.

"The hormones in the Pill may interfere with the surges of estrogen that you get during exercise that help build bone," says lead researcher Connie Weaver, PhD, head of the department of foods and nutrition at the university. "Adequate calcium seems to offset that."

How much calcium do you need? While *Prevention* recommends 1,000 mg per day for most women in the 18-to-30 range, exercisers on the Pill may need 1,200 mg per day to preserve precious bone density.

once a week. Because Fosamax isn't easily absorbed, up until now it had to be taken each morning with 8 oz water on an empty stomach. For a full half hour after taking it, you couldn't eat, drink, or even lie down. If you didn't follow these rules, the drug could come back up into your esophagus and cause pain and discomfort.

But now the FDA has approved a once-a-week dose of Fosamax. Studies show it to be as effective as the daily dose, and it has fewer side effects. You still have to follow the "no food, no drinking, no lying down" rules of the daily regi-men, but only once a week. "It's wonderful. I almost never use the daily formulation anymore. The once-weekly regimen is so much easier and fits in with my philosophy about pills: The fewer, the better," says Dr. Cosman.

What to do: Ask your doctor for the once-a-week dose of Fosamax. But if you are happy with your daily routine, you don't have to change. Another choice: a nasal spray (Miacalcin). It's fuss-free but somewhat less effective than bisphospho-nates. Another option for postmenopausal women is hormone replacement therapy.

New Secrets for Stronger Bones

You already know that weight lifting strengthens bones. But now we know which exercises work best to stop bone loss and whether weight loss can harm your bones.

Researchers at the University of Arizona in Tucson examined 266 postmenopausal women for a full year. Half of them did resistance and weight bearing exercises; all were taking calci-um supplements. Here's what the results showed that you should do.

Ponder HRT and exercise. Sure, your bones are better off if you exercise than if you don't. They're also better off if you take hormone replacement therapy (HRT) than if you don't. But the women who are best off are those who do *both*. If you're wondering which works better, it's a tie. Exercise was better at strengthening the hipbone, but HRT worked better on the spine. Incidentally, the combination of HRT, exercise, and calcium supplemen-tation looks like the best bet of all.

Do your squats. Some bones proved more responsive to exercise than others. Why? "It's probably due to the types of exercises done," says study author and physiology profes-sor Tim Lohman, PhD. In particular, squats and leg presses have a strong impact on the hip area, whereas it's harder to strengthen the spine through exercise.

Also, the more weight the women lifted, the greater the hip benefited—which is tremendously important, because it's the bone most prone to fractures. A routine of two sets of six to eight reps is recommended, and the weight you lift should be heavy enough so the last two or three repetitions are tough. See p. 54 for more on performing squats correctly.

You think you're using all available treatments to protect your bones.

What your doctor needs to know: A powerful new treatment called injectable parathyroid hormone (PTH) could be available by the end of this year and could be one of the most dramatic advances in osteoporosis treatment in recent history. "This may become one of the first drugs approved by the FDA that builds bone," says John Bilezikian, MD, director of the metabolic bone diseases program at Columbia–Presbyterian Medical Center in New York City.

In a study of 1,637 postmenopausal women at Massachusetts General Hospital in Boston, women treated with injectable PTH for about 18 months increased bone mass up to 13% in the spine and reduced their risk of fractures by 69%.

Your body already makes PTH, which helps regulate blood and bone calcium levels and keeps the bone-forming system active and on track. Researchers first discovered the potential of PTH as a bone-building treatment when they found

Aim for some impact. If you've been walking in the hopes that it will build bone, we've got some interesting news. While walking does help *maintain* bone mass, it doesn't help build it or prevent bone loss. To build bone, you'll need to also do some weight training and/or some moderate or high-impact activities such as jogging, running, or jumping rope. See "The Run-Walk Program" on p. 62 for a safe way to add some speedwork to your walking routine.

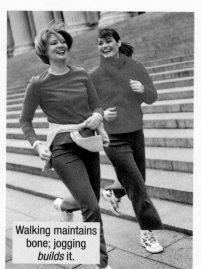

Walking maintains bone; jogging *builds* it.

Maintain your weight. If you're already in a healthy range, don't lose more weight. Though we don't know exactly why, women who lost more than 10 lb of body weight lost bone density as well. There may be a relationship between fat loss and bone loss, but more research is needed to find out why. The good news: Those who slimmed down but were on HRT still gained bone mass.

Stay emotionally fit. The women with the highest vitality enjoyed the most benefit to their bones. Depression, which is known to alter body chemistry, appeared to have a negative effect in building bone strength.

Eat all the essentials. Calcium isn't the only nutrient essential for strong bones. Though we need more research to identify other specific bone-building nutrients, the women in this study who ate the healthiest, most well-rounded diets benefited more in bone health, says Dr. Lohman.

that people who make too much PTH had relatively healthy spinal bone densities. They also theorized that postmenopausal women may experience a loss of sensitivity to their own PTH system—in addition to estrogen loss at menopause that could account for the decrease in bone mass and development of osteoporosis that they experience, adds Dr. Bilezikian.

The FDA is currently reviewing the drug for approval. If it's approved, you'd take a daily dose through an injection pen, much like the one people with diabetes use to inject insulin.

There could be even more good news about PTH. Dr. Bilezikian and his associates are now

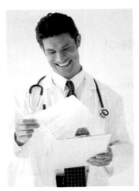

Ask your doctor to keep on top of new advances in bone protection.

conducting a study supplementing PTH with bone-preserving drugs, also known as anti-resorptives, to prevent bone loss. Concerns about over-stimulating bone growth with PTH means that you may only be able to take it for 1 to 2 years, so researchers want to know if anti-resorptive drugs will preserve PTH-related bone density gains. Dr. Bilezikian is also investigating the effects of using PTH and anti-resorptive drugs at the same time. He expects results within 2 years.

What to do: Ask your doctor to keep track of FDA approval as well as further studies on combining PTH with drugs such as Fosamax.

Your Family Medical History
Answer these questions today to help ensure a healthier future

Recording a detailed family medical history can be a lifesaving project for you and your loved ones. Try to collect the information below for each member of four generations: you, your children, your siblings and their children, your parents, your mom's and dad's parents, and your aunts, uncles, and cousins. (You'll want to make plenty of extra copies of this page first!)

If you have kids, gather the same information for your spouse's family. If you can't obtain all of the information, don't worry; your doctor will work with you to determine what information is necessary.

Name/Relationship _____

Date of Birth _____

Lifestyle and Habits

▶ Smoking _____

_____

▶ Alcohol use _____

▶ Recreational drug use _____

_____

▶ Obesity _____

_____

Notes: _____

_____

Medications _____

_____

Allergies _____

_____

Also see your notes on your reproductive history on p. 153.

Specific Medical Problems (Include age at time of diagnosis)

▶ Number of cancers _____

▶ Original sites of cancers _____

▶ Areas to which cancer spread _____

▶ Heart disease _____

▶ High blood pressure _____

▶ High cholesterol _____

▶ High triglycerides _____

▶ Diabetes _____

▶ Alzheimer's disease _____

▶ Osteoporosis _____

▶ Depression _____

▶ Other illnesses _____

▶ Major surgeries _____

Notes: _____

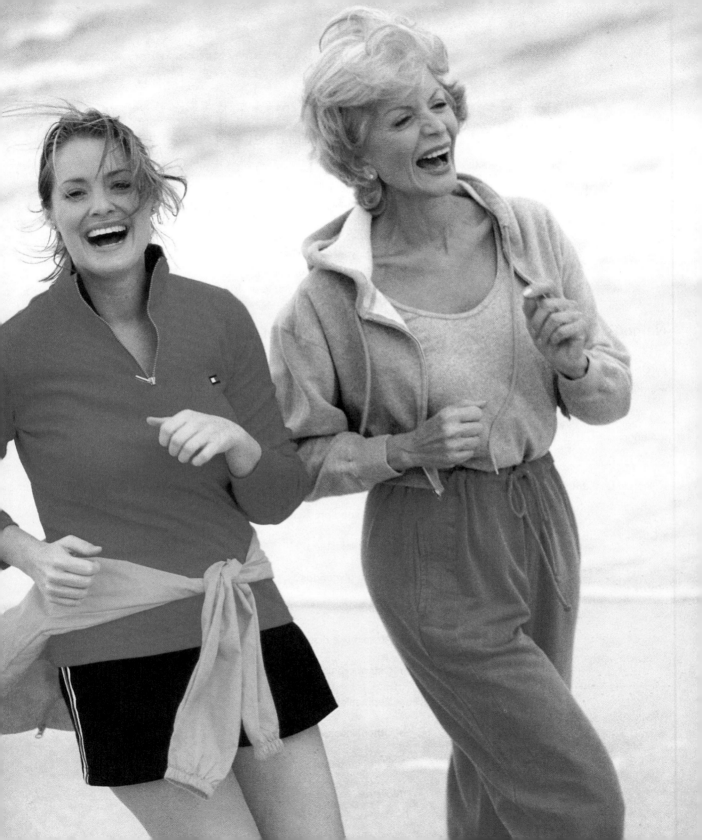

PART FOUR

Mammograms, Menopause, and More

CHAPTER 17

The Truth about Mammograms

Prevention advisor Mary Jane Minkin, MD, cuts through the confusion and controversy

The question of whether or not women should get mammograms—and how often—isn't as simple as you might think.

Prevention has long recommended that all women over 40 get a mammogram each year—and still does. But in the early 2000s, some seemingly contradictory studies came out, clouding the issue and confusing plenty of women. If you're among the women wondering whether this test is worth the time and money, you'll want to take the time to read this chapter from start to finish. In the past 3 years, additional research has been done to determine whether or not mammograms are important. Here's what you need to know to make an informed decision about this lifesaving test, based on the latest research.

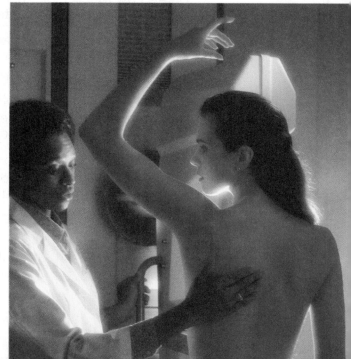

Mammograms catch cancer earlier than self-exams do.

The Science behind Mammograms

Historically, clinical trials have shown that if you're a woman in your 40s, regular mammograms can reduce your chances of dying from breast cancer by about 17%. If you're between 50 and 69, they showed that you can reduce your risk by 30%. Then in 2001, a new study from Sweden made those numbers—which are pretty significant—pale by comparison. Their results showed that regular mammograms can actually reduce the risk of breast cancer death by more than 60%!

Why were the numbers so different from those of previous studies? It was largely a difference in how the studies were done. In the previous studies, half of the women were assigned to a group that was "invited" to get a mammogram—but not all of them did. And sometimes women from the "non-mammogram" group got mammograms anyway. The result? When experts compared the breast cancer deaths of both groups, the women who didn't stick to the program led to an underestimation of the true benefit of mammography screenings.

That's why Swedish researchers did a *new* study—to get a truer picture of the impact of regular mammography. This study compared breast cancer deaths in women ages 40 to 69 (during a time when mammograms weren't available in two Swedish counties) with deaths among women who were offered mammograms every 2 years (when organized community screening subsequently became policy).

The results were pretty astounding. Breast cancer deaths were 63% lower among the women who took advantage of the screenings than among those women for whom mammography was not yet available. "As our study shows, the woman who gets a mammogram on a regular basis reduces her risk of dying from breast cancer by about two-thirds," says Robert A. Smith, PhD, director of cancer screening for the American Cancer Society in Atlanta and coauthor of the study.

DO JUST ONE THING!

Move to Beat Breast Cancer

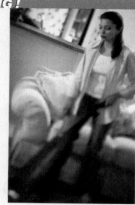

Clean up—and cut your cancer risk!

Whether you vacuum, wait tables, or jog, if you get some form of exercise, you're beating your breast cancer odds, according to Canadian researchers. Scientists surveyed 2,470 women—half with breast cancer and half without. They discovered that postmenopausal women who did the greatest amount of moderate activity (such as cleaning or assembly work) throughout their life had a 30% lower risk of breast cancer than those who did the least.

For the best protection, aim for both moderate and vigorous activity (such as jogging or another type of aerobic workout) most days. Researchers speculate that activity protects you by lowering your levels of high-risk hormones as well as by preventing weight gain, which is a risk factor for breast cancer.

How much of the improvement in the survival rate in the screened group is due to improved treatment of breast cancer? "There's no question that treatment has contributed something," explains Dr. Smith. "But overwhelmingly, the critical factor in survival from breast cancer is the size of the tumor when the cancer is diagnosed. Mammography enables the cancer to be discovered when it is at an earlier stage."

‖ The Controversy

Unfortunately, around the same time that the Swedish study was published, *The Lancet* published a letter in which two Danish researchers restated the original conclusion of a paper they published in 2000; it said that mammograms are "unjustified," because there is no reliable evidence that they save lives.

In their original paper, these Danish researchers analyzed seven randomized trials of mammography screening published in the 1980s and 1990s and concluded that it doesn't save lives. (They didn't do new research, but simply reanalyzed existing study information.) Five of the studies from their analysis were discarded right off the bat, because they were judged to be of poor quality or extremely flawed.

At the time that the analysis was published, it was discredited for being flawed in its own right. "The Danish researchers made any number of arbitrary decisions and arguable judgments about the quality of the trials," explains Dr. Smith. They were very critical of studies that were favorable toward mammography and very accepting of studies that showed no benefit for mammography, according to Dr. Smith. The researchers based their conclusion on two studies alone, which is "just a fraction of the existing world data," adds Dr. Smith.

Given all the criticism, in 2001, the Danish researchers reanalyzed their findings. To no one's surprise, they stood by their original conclusion.

1-MINUTE *HEALTH BOOSTER*

Talk Yourself into a Mammogram

In spite of all the convincing data and public health messages about the importance of mammograms, only 50 to 60% of American women get tested regularly. If you're skipping this test because of fear, try these tips to talk yourself into getting this important screening.

▶ Remind yourself that a mammogram can provide reassurance that you don't have breast cancer.

▶ Ask a girlfriend to go with you when you have your mammogram. Better yet, schedule your mammograms together, and enjoy lunch afterward.

▶ Remember that it's never too late to start having regular mammograms.

▶ Have someone schedule the appointment for you, if necessary.

▶ Cut back on caffeine for 2 to 4 weeks before your next mammogram; it may help reduce mammogram discomfort.

This is what made news and led to the latest controversy about mammograms' effectiveness.

What most people didn't realize, however, was that this letter did not contain any new research findings and was based on their highly criticized original paper.

What *You* Need to Know

"If you approach the issue from a scientific perspective, it's clearly settled," according to Daniel B. Kopans, MD, professor of radiology at Harvard Medical School. If you look at all of the randomized controlled trials, there is a 25 to 30% statistically significant mortality reduction with mammography screening. In addition, many other studies show that mammography finds breast cancers when they're smaller and at an earlier stage, which we know translates into better survival. "In my opinion, these data have not been refuted by the Danish researchers. They just choose not to believe them," Dr. Kopans adds.

The death rate from breast cancer has been steadily dropping by 1 to 2% a year since around 1990. That's what you'd expect to see given that mammography screening became more widespread in the US during the mid-1980s—and breast cancer therapy became more effective.

There's no dispute about the value of mammograms, according to Dr. Smith. Women should continue to have confidence in the judgment of numerous US and European groups that have reached a very different conclusion from the Danish researchers. "Mammography won't save everyone's life, but as the Swedish study demonstrated,

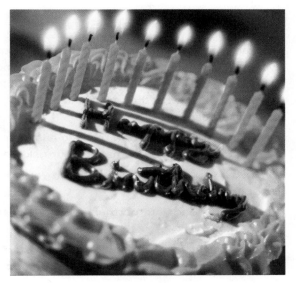

Use your birthday as a reminder to schedule your annual mammogram.

it provides the opportunity to reduce the death rate by as much as 63%—twice the benefit than previously estimated," says Dr. Kopans.

Still the Best Early Detector

Mammograms are still the best way to find cancer at its earliest stage. "Four years ago, the average size of a breast cancer detected was 2 centimeters, or about 1". Now it is below 1 centimeter," says Amy Langer, executive director of the National Alliance of Breast Cancer Organizations in New York City and a 17-year breast cancer survivor. Langer attributes this to early

Anxiety-Free Self-Exams

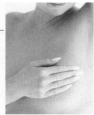

Exams *can* be easy.

If examining your breasts monthly for suspicious lumps makes you nervous, you're in good company. A new UCLA study finds that women at higher risk of breast cancer are less likely to perform this potentially lifesaving test because they're afraid of what they might find. If you're among them, try these tips for reducing breast self-exam jitters.

1. Ask your doctor for a realistic assessment of your breast cancer odds. You could be overestimating your risk, causing yourself undue anxiety.

2. Ask your gynecologist to teach you how to do a thorough breast self-exam.

3. Bring along your partner, if you'd like, so that you can learn to do the exam together.

4. Examine your breasts 2 to 3 days after the end of your menstrual period, when you have the least amount of swelling from fluid retention.

detection and the vastly improved quality of mammograms today.

Finding breast cancer early also affects your treatment choices. If a doctor can detect a tumor at an earlier stage, when it can be treated with a lumpectomy rather than mastectomy or when a patient won't need radiation or chemotherapy, that can make a huge difference in her life.

The debate about mammography may never be settled to everyone's satisfaction. In the meantime, urges Langer, don't forgo the opportunity to have the biggest edge against breast cancer you can by doing what is within your control. "You can't pick your genes or your parents, but you can do everything in your power to make sure you find breast cancer if it's there."

Prevention isn't changing its mammogram screening recommendations:

▶ Have a mammogram every year if you are age 40 or older.

▶ Have a clinical breast exam every year by a health care professional who is well trained in doing breast exams and performs them on a regular basis.

▶ Practice monthly breast self-examination. (See "Anxiety-Free Self-Exams" above for helpful advice on this topic.)

If your insurance doesn't cover a screening mammogram, call the American Cancer Society at (800) ACS-2345 (227-2345) or the Centers for Disease Control and Prevention toll-free at (888) 842-6355 for information on getting a free or low-cost mammogram.

CHAPTER 18

Honest Answers to Common Questions

Straight talk about birth control, menopause, and more

Every month, women write to *Prevention* with important questions about uniquely female concerns. In this chapter, we share some of the most common, along with smart advice from *Prevention* advisor Mary Jane Minkin, MD, a board-certified obstetrician-gynecologist in New Haven, CT, clinical professor at Yale University School of Medicine, and coauthor of *What Every Woman Needs to Know about Menopause* (Yale University Press, 1996).

While we've tried to cover topics that you'll find interesting, you may find yourself coming up with additional questions about reproductive health. To make sure you don't forget to address them during your next yearly exam, jot them down on p. 152, then take this book along to your doctor visit.

Got questions?
Your doctor should
be happy to help.

‖ Pap Test Update

My gynecologist asked if I wanted a ThinPrep Pap test. What is that—and why would I want one?

ThinPrep helps avoid repeat Paps.

The conventional method for Pap testing involves collecting a sample of cervical cells—often accompanied by blood, mucus, and other debris—and smearing it on a slide for examination at a lab. With the Thin-Prep method, which has been around since the late '90s, the instrument used to collect the cells is "rinsed" into a container of liquid. When it reaches the lab, a special process separates the cervical cells from the debris, then applies a thin layer of cells to a slide. Here are a few of the benefits of ThinPrep:

▶ Research suggests that ThinPrep results in higher quality slides that are easier for technicians to read.

▶ Studies show that ThinPrep results in fewer unsatisfactory or limited slides that would require a repeat Pap.

▶ Preliminary data indicates that ThinPrep may even pick up more glandular lesions (adenocarcinoma) than the traditional Pap test—a rarer type of cancer than squamous cell cancer. (In theory, it should also be better at picking up squamous cell cancer, although research has not yet proven that.)

ThinPrep is not the only liquid-based test, but it is the most widely used. For the above reasons, you may choose to go with this method if it is offered. If, however, your doctor doesn't offer ThinPrep, the traditional Pap is still an excellent test, so don't be concerned. Having a yearly Pap test of *either* type is the best thing you can do to eliminate your risk for cervical cancer.

‖ More Convenient Birth Control

I have been wanting to switch from the Pill to a more convenient form of birth control. How do patches and contraceptive rings rate?

While it's hard to top the Pill for effectiveness, both patches and rings may top it for convenience. Here's the lowdown on each, but be sure you discuss all of your options with your gynecologist before switching birth control methods.

Contraceptive patch. Clinical studies show the patch to be as effective as the low-dose Pill in preventing pregnancy, but it eliminates the daily pill-taking routine. The patch, sold under the name Ortho Evra, combines low-dose estrogen and a progestin in a 1¾" square transdermal patch that you wear on your upper arm, abdomen, back, or buttocks. The patch is replaced every 7 days for 3 consecutive weeks. The fourth week of your cycle is patch-free (when you have your period).

The once-a-week contraception solution.

Contraceptive ring. NuvaRing became the first contraceptive vaginal ring when it was approved by the FDA in 2001. A flexible 2" round ring, it compresses for easy insertion into your vagina. NuvaRing releases a low dose of estrogen and progestin into the surrounding tissue, so you

The ring offers 3-week protection.

need less of the two hormones than you would if you took birth control pills.

The ring stays in place for 3 weeks. It's removed for the fourth week of the menstrual cycle, after which a new ring is inserted. Like the Pill and the patch, it works by preventing ovulation.

Menopause and the Pill

"Since the Pill is keeping my periods regular, how will I know if I'm nearing menopause?"

The first clue for most women that they're peri-menopausal (in the transition to menopause) is that their menstrual cycles become irregular or their flow may be lighter or heavier than usual. But because birth control pills are so good at reg-ulating the menstrual cycle, you won't have the benefit of these changes to help guide you. Watch for these signs instead.

Look for symptoms during the week you're off the Pill and taking the placebo pills. During this part of your cycle, you may begin to experience symptoms such as hot flashes, night sweats, insomnia, or even headaches. These signs of estrogen withdrawal occur because you're not getting estrogen this week, and your body's own estrogen levels are fluctuating.

Look at your family history. How old was your mother when she first began to approach began menopause? This can be a reliable predictor of when you will go through it, provided that hers was a natural menopause and not the result of a hysterectomy.

Consider your age. The average age of menopause in the US is 51. The true sign that you've officially reached menopause is when you've gone without a period for 12 consecutive months. The only way to know this for certain is

Don't Automatically Self-Treat Infections

When you have a vaginal infection, don't assume it's yeast-based. The culprit could be an equally common vaginal infection called bacterial vaginosis, or BV.

How can you tell which is which? BV is caused by a disruption of the normal balance between good and bad bacteria in the vagina—not by an overgrowth of yeast. Anything that alters the vaginal pH, such as antibiotics or douching, can trigger this.

BV typically has a fishy odor and a thin, milky white or gray discharge. There may or may not be itching and burning. With a yeast infection, however, there is no odor, the discharge is "cottage-cheesy," and there is almost always vaginal itching and burning.

To diagnose BV, your health care provider will examine you for signs of irritation, inflamma-tion, and discharge, which she will take a sample of and test.

Why is it so important to see your doctor for a diagnosis? Left untreated, BV can cause serious health problems such as pelvic inflammatory disease, increased risk of STDs, and pregnancy complications.

Learn about Fibroids

Between 25 and 35% of women have fibroids. You could be one and not even realize it, since they never cause problems for most women who have them.

What are fibroids? Fibroids—also called leiomyomas—are benign overgrowths of the layer of muscle tissue that comprises the uterus. They can range in size from a pea to a cantaloupe.

What causes fibroids to grow? Fibroids depend on estrogen for growth, which is why they're more common in women in their 40s when hormonal changes begin to occur prior to menopause. This is also the time when they can cause symptoms. Fortunately, fibroids shrink after menopause (unless you take estrogen replacement therapy).

What symptoms do fibroids cause? For 10 to 20% of women with fibroids, symptoms may include heavy menstrual bleeding, pelvic pain and pressure, frequent urination, and abdominal distention. If you have any of these symptoms, call your doctor right away, since these symptoms may also indicate other serious health problems. Your doctor can best diagnose you and recommend an appropriate course of action.

to stop taking birth control pills. (Be sure to use another form of birth control in the meantime.) Note: If you're a smoker, you may go through menopause even earlier. Smoking can accelerate menopause by about 2 years due to the toxic effect it has on the ovaries.

Consider having your level of follicle-stimulating hormone (FSH) measured with a blood test. As your ovaries stop making as much estrogen, your pituitary gland responds with a burst of FSH to tell the ovaries to increase estrogen production. A woman's FSH levels can fluctuate enormously during perimenopause, so your doctor will likely take several readings over time. A high FSH (one that falls in the range of 40 to 50 mIU/ml), especially if you're having hot flashes or night sweats, could mean you're headed in the direction of menopause.

When the Bottom Drops Out

"I get a feeling of heaviness in my vaginal area, and sometimes it feels like my insides are dropping. What's going on here?"

From your symptoms, you likely have some degree of pelvic floor relaxation, which goes by the fancy name of *pelvic organ prolapse*. This doesn't automatically mean that you need surgery. In fact, a little muscle rehab may be enough to relieve your symptoms.

What may be happening: Normally, an assortment of muscles, ligaments, connective tissue, and nerves all work together to support your pelvic organs, which include your bladder, uterus, vagina, and rectum. If the muscles become weak, or the ligaments and tissues become stretched or damaged, any one of these organs can drop down and press against the walls of the vagina.

The result is the feeling of heaviness or the sensation that things are "dropping out." Some women may have a pulling sensation or achiness in their pelvic area, leak urine, or have trouble moving their bowels. If the prolapse is severe enough, the pelvic organs can bulge into the walls of the vagina, causing tissue to protrude through your vaginal opening.

What may have caused it: Pelvic organ prolapse is almost exclusively a female health problem and one that affects many women. The additional weight a woman carries when she is pregnant, along with the stresses of labor and vaginal delivery, can leave the ligaments and muscles stretched and weak. Even if you haven't had children, the loss of estrogen at menopause as well as normal aging can cause the pelvic tissues to weaken.

What you can do: See your gynecologist for a thorough pelvic exam if you suspect you have pelvic organ prolapse. This condition can worsen over time. The sooner you learn the extent of your problem, the sooner you can take steps to remedy it.

If your doctor isn't familiar with pelvic organ prolapse, find one who diagnoses and treats it as part of their daily practice. And always seek a second opinion before agreeing to any type of surgery to correct the problem. Often, physical therapy of the pelvic floor, along with a pessary (a removable ring-like device that props up pelvic organs), is enough to provide relief—although for some women, surgery *is* the most effective treatment.

Prevent Pelvic Floor Problems

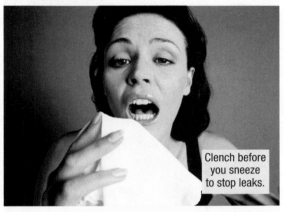

Clench before you sneeze to stop leaks.

You can try to avoid pelvic organ prolapse by keeping your pelvic floor muscles in good shape with these tips:

▶ **Lose excess weight.**

▶ **Don't smoke.**

▶ **Avoid constipation and straining with bowel movements.**

▶ **Avoid constant heavy lifting.**

▶ **Get a chronic cough due to allergies under control.**

▶ **Practice Kegel exercises regularly. (Have your health care provider instruct you on technique and frequency.)**

▶ **After pregnancy and delivery, be alert for signs that you've lost some pelvic support. Early muscle rehab can minimize your problems down the road.**

▶ **And just before you sneeze, jump, or lift something heavy, tighten your pelvic muscles, and hold them until you're finished.**

CHAPTER 19

Are Those Menopause Symptoms...or Worse?

Here's how to tell if your hot flashes and skipped periods indicate a life-threatening health condition

It's easy to assume that every change your body undergoes after the age of 40 is a merely another sign that menopause is on its way. And it's even easier to make that assumption when your doctor seems to agree. "When a woman is of the right age for menopause, there's almost a knee-jerk reaction on the part of doctors to attribute any symptom to menopause and not investigate other causes," says James A. Simon, MD, clinical professor of obstetrics and gynecology at The George Washington University School of Medicine and Health Sciences in Washington, DC.

This "go home, it's just menopause" response is all too common when it comes to women 40 to 60, according to Marianne J. Legato, MD, founder and director of the Partnership for Women's Health at

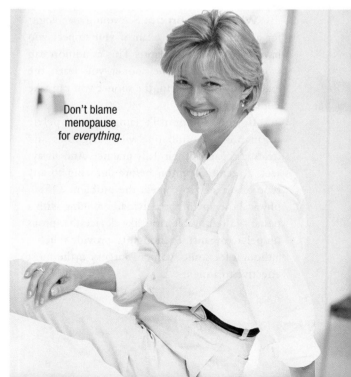

Don't blame menopause for *everything*.

Columbia University in New York City. "Dismissing or minimizing women's complaints as menopause or 'it's all in your head' puts them at risk for a serious underlying condition going undiagnosed," explains Dr. Legato.

Here's a look at six familiar symptoms associated with menopause and how to know when you and your doctor should take a closer look at them.

1. Changes in Periods

Irregular menstrual periods—one of the most common and predictable signs of menopause—most often occur because of the erratic levels of estrogen and progesterone and less-frequent ovulation. "Irregular" means periods with bleeding that is lighter or heavier than usual, periods that are closer together, bleeding for fewer or more days than usual, or periods that are skipped altogether.

It may be menopause, but it could be . . .

a hormone imbalance, thyroid disease, uterine fibroids (enlarged by the surge of estrogen as you approach menopause), uterine polyps (noncancerous growths in the endometrium), or even cervical or uterine cancer. All of these can cause menstrual irregularities, which is why it's important that you see your doctor if your periods start to change.

Getting the right diagnosis is crucial if you want to avoid unnecessary procedures such as a hysterectomy, says Michelle Warren, MD, medical director of the Center for Menopause, Hormonal Disorders, and Women's Health at Columbia University in New York City.

Here's what you should do.

Menstrual changes that are considered abnormal and need to be checked out by your doctor include the following:

▶ Periods that are very heavy and gushing, or bleeding with clots
▶ Periods that last more than 7 days
▶ Periods that last 2 or more days longer than usual
▶ Spotting between periods
▶ Bleeding after intercourse
▶ Fewer than 21 days between periods

Your doctor will want to know what triggers the bleeding and what makes it stop. Tests used to help determine the cause of abnormal bleeding include a Pap test; a transvaginal ultrasound (which uses sound waves to visualize the uterus and other pelvic organs with a probe inserted into the vagina); endometrial biopsy (in which a small sample of the uterine lining is removed and examined); or hysteroscopy (where a tiny telescope is inserted into the vagina and through the cervix to look directly at the uterine lining).

Irregular periods may signal menopause . . .
or thyroid disease . . . or fibroids . . . or even cervical cancer.
Let your doctor be the judge.

2. Hot Flashes and Night Sweats

Hot flashes or flushes are the second most frequent symptom associated with menopause. When they occur with often-drenching perspiration during the night, they're called night sweats.

Hot flashes are the body's way of cooling itself down. Abrupt changes in the body's "thermostat" in the brain can cause it to mistakenly sense that you're too warm. So blood vessels dilate, and blood rushes to the surface of the skin to cool the body. That's why you get the red, flushed look on your face and neck. Sweating, which sometimes accompanies a hot flash, also cools the body as the perspiration evaporates.

It may be menopause, but it could be . . .

Hyperthyroidism. That's because the symptoms of an overactive thyroid—which can include flushing, sweating, heat intolerance, heart palpitations, and sleeplessness—can easily be confused with those of menopause. If left untreated, an overactive thyroid can cause a loss of bone mineral density, which, over time, can lead to osteoporosis. Hyperthyroidism can also result in an irregular heartbeat, which can lead to stroke or heart failure.

An infectious disease. If you're feeling sick in addition to experiencing hot flashes and sweating, you could have an infectious disease such as tuberculosis, Lyme disease, or AIDS. "When you're having menopausal hot flashes, you may feel tired because you haven't had a good night's sleep, but you shouldn't feel sick," says Dr. Simon.

Certain cancers. Sweating along with a fever could also be caused by cancers such as leukemia or lymphomas. A rare tumor of the adrenal gland called a pheochromocytoma and one that usually occurs in the intestine called a carcinoid tumor can cause flushing and feelings of warmth too, which could be mistaken for menopause symptoms.

Here's what you should do.

If you're losing weight but not dieting, your heart frequently beats rapidly, you're always hot even when people around you are cold, you feel generally unwell, or you have a fever, don't ignore it. A blood test called a TSH (thyroid-stimulating hormone) test can tell your doctor if the culprit is hyperthyroidism, and other tests can be run to rule out infection or cancer. Even if menopause truly *is* to blame, you'll feel better knowing that you've checked out all of the possibilities.

3. Hair Loss

"Once a day, I hear 'I'm losing my hair. Is it menopause?'" says Mary Jane Minkin, MD, *Prevention* advisor and a clinical professor of obstetrics and gynecology at Yale University School of Medicine. There may well be a connection between dwindling estrogen levels at menopause and thinning hair, but there's no conclusive data.

It may be menopause, but it could be . . .

Hypothyroidism. Thyroid changes—even subtle ones—can affect hair. Complaints of dry skin or brittle nails are also common in women with underactive thyroids. Other symptoms of an underactive thyroid also can be easily mistaken for signs of menopause: heavy menstrual bleeding, fatigue, painful joints, mood swings, and weight

1-MINUTE *HEALTH BOOSTER*

Tune Out Joint Pain

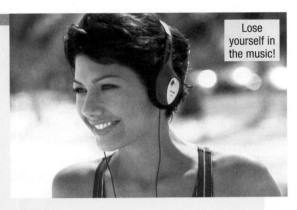

Lose yourself in the music!

If your joint pain turns out to be a result of rheumatoid arthritis (an autoimmune disease of the joints that causes pain and swelling), don't rule out the possibility of continuing to exercise regularly. Working out is often exactly what doctors recommend to improve mobility. How to prevent pain from sidelining you? Move to some music, say experts.

In a small study at Glasgow University in Scotland, researchers found that women with rheumatoid arthritis could walk 30% farther when they listened to music of their choice than when they walked in silence. "The music didn't make their pain disappear," says lead researcher Paul MacIntyre, MD. "It took their mind off it, so they could walk farther without needing to stop." As a bonus, regular exercise can help ease midlife stresses that many women face around the time of menopause, including caring for aging parents and raising teenagers.

gain. If hypothyroidism is not treated, it can raise your cholesterol and increase your risk of heart disease. It can also lead to a decline in memory and concentration.

Here's what you should do.

Ask for a TSH test. That way, you can avoid being given a prescription for estrogen replacement therapy, when you really need a prescription for thyroid hormone.

4. Achy Joints

Joint pain and stiffness are common but not well-recognized symptoms of menopause, says Dr. Warren, because studies have not found a direct link between achy joints and the "change of life."

Usually the joint pain and stiffness associated with menopause isn't localized to a specific joint but is described more as an overall achiness. The pain or stiffness also doesn't "migrate," or show up in your elbow one day and your knee the next.

It may be menopause, but it could be . . .

Osteoarthritis. Pain in key joints such as the hips, knees, lower back, or end joints of the fingers is most likely not menopause but osteoarthritis. "Osteoarthritis has a pattern to it, so you'll have pain or stiffness when you get up in the morning or after using a joint for a long period of time," explains John Klippel, MD, medical director of the Arthritis Foundation in Atlanta.

We know that a lack of estrogen affects bone

and probably cartilage, according to Dr. Klippel. That could explain why osteoarthritis affects mostly women and typically begins when they're in their mid-to-late 40s.

Here's what you should do.

See a doctor if your joint pain persists or is accompanied by swelling, or if you have difficulty using the joint. Other types of arthritis should also be ruled out, such as rheumatoid arthritis, fibromyalgia, lupus, or Lyme disease.

5. Depression

We know from studies that giving estrogen to women during perimenopause (the transition to menopause) helps reduce their depression. Other studies have suggested that estrogen improves mood in postmenopausal women who feel depressed.

Depression may also be triggered by the loss of sleep that hot flashes and night sweats can cause. Sleep problems can leave you feeling irritable, which may result in the loss of your overall sense of well-being.

All of this doesn't mean that depression is inevitable at menopause, but when it does occur, it should be taken seriously and investigated. Women with a history of depression seem to be more vulnerable to depression at menopause, so they should be especially vigilant for its symptoms.

It may be menopause, but it could be . . .

Hypothyroidism. Since depression is also a symptom of this thyroid imbalance, make sure you've ruled out this condition with a TSH test.

Stress. Caring for aging parents, raising teenagers, career changes, or financial problems often hit at this time and can affect anyone's abil-

Ease Stress, Sleep Better

Anywhere from 23 to 42% of women experience trouble sleeping during the menopause transition. Sometimes hormonal fluctuations are to blame, but often anxiety plays a role too. If your doctor believes that stress is keeping you up nights, try these tips for bringing your life into balance.

Keep a worry journal. Choose a time during the day when you can write down worries and concerns, along with potential solutions. If you take time to deal with your stresses during the day, they're less likely to plague you at night.

Exercise regularly. Just make sure that you do so at least 2 to 3 hours *before* bedtime so you have time to wind down.

Try yoga or tai chi. Both are gentle forms of exercise that encourage you to slow down and relax.

Get organized before bed. Planning out the following day may help clear your mind before you go to sleep.

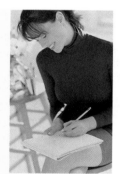

Put your fears on paper.

ity to cope. A good assessment by your physician and some soul-searching on your part may reveal that speaking with a mental health professional would be much more beneficial than estrogen therapy.

Here's what you should do.

Symptoms that go beyond normal feelings of sadness, such as significant changes in weight, social withdrawal, disinterest in life, insomnia, inability to concentrate, and anxiety, should never be dismissed. You could be experiencing a clinical depression, which is best treated with a combination of medication and psychotherapy.

6. Palpitations

Palpitations can feel like the heart is beating erratically or fast, or skipping a beat, or as if there are butterflies in your chest. Usually they occur with hot flashes and night sweats, but they can appear on their own.

"Levels of estrogen during perimenopause alternate between very high and very low," says Dr. Legato. "This causes a destabilization of the cardiac rhythm, which can lead to palpitations." If it turns out that your palpitations are related to menopause, they can usually be relieved with estrogen replacement therapy.

It may be menopause, but it could be . . .

Hyperthyroidism. A revved-up thyroid can increase the effects of adrenaline, a stress hormone in the body, which can cause a rapid heart rhythm or arrhythmia. It's diagnosed with a TSH test.

A serious heart rhythm abnormality or heart disease. Palpitations that occur in

DO JUST ONE THING!
Ask for a TSH Test

Women between the ages of 30 and 50 are most typically affected with hypothyroidism (an underactive thyroid), and it's estimated that 10% of women 40 and older go undiagnosed. This is one of the reasons that the American Association of Clinical Endocrinologists recommends that all women over the age of 40 have a TSH (thyroid-stimulating hormone) test.

TSH, which is made by the pituitary gland, regulates the amount of thyroid hormone that is released into the blood. A TSH blood test can determine whether you have an overactive or underactive thyroid, both of which can cause symptoms similar to those associated with menopause.

the absence of hot flashes on a recurring basis or are associated with light-headedness or shortness of breath warrant a cardiac evaluation.

Here's what you should do.

See your doctor, and be sure he runs tests to rule out both thyroid and cardiac problems.

One cardiac test that can be done is an electrocardiogram, called an EKG or ECG, which measures the electrical impulses of the heart and can show an irregularity in the heartbeat.

A stress echocardiogram is also a very accurate method of diagnosing heart disease in women. It's an imaging technique, which combines a treadmill stress test with cardiac ultrasound to check your heart's size, movement, shape, and pumping ability.

CHAPTER 20

Do-It-Yourself Menopause Remedies

Herbalist Aviva Romm's all-natural tonics for hot flashes, mood swings, and more

Adult women all know that we're someday destined for menopause. And while we may welcome the end to menstruation, none of us is thrilled with the hot flashes, night sweats, insomnia, memory glitches, and mood swings that mark the transition to our period-free years. For some women, hormone replacement therapy (HRT) is a good solution to minimizing the symptoms of this transition. But not every woman can take HRT, and even if you *can,* that doesn't mean it's your only option.

If you're among the women who would prefer to try herbal and dietary measures to minimize the symptoms of menopause, then you'll love this chapter, written by Aviva Romm, certified professional midwife and professional member of the American Herbalists Guild (AHG). Romm, an

Relax! Mother Nature knows how to handle menopause!

herbalist and midwife for 15 years, is the executive director of the AHG and the director of LifeCycles Midwifery and Herbal Medicine in Canton, GA. On the pages that follow, you'll find her recommendations for managing menopause naturally.

Aviva's Herbal Menopause Remedies

Over the past 15 years, I've developed a variety of herbal formulas that effectively relieve menopausal symptoms for many of the women I've treated. Some are delicious teas; others are blends of liquid extracts.

In some of the formulas, I recommend using tinctures, which are liquid herbal extracts, because I believe they act more quickly, are more potent, and generally offer better results than capsules. If you don't like their taste, try diluting tinctures in a little fruit juice. These doses are appropriate for tinctures in 1:3, 1:4, and 1:5 concentrations.

You can find most of these herbs at health food stores; increasingly, herbs are sold at pharmacies and even supermarkets. Choose only single-herb products. Some formulas take time to work, so in order to feel better, you must take them for as long as indicated in their directions. For all remedies, when a range of doses is noted, start with the smallest dose, and increase only if necessary.

DO JUST ONE THING!

Know Your Menopause Herbs

Here, Douglas Schar, DipPhyt, MCPP, MNIMH, a European-trained clinical herbalist, explains the specific benefits of five of the major menopause-relief herbs found in the remedies in this chapter.

Black cohosh. Reduces the severity of hot flashes, memory loss, depression, and mood swings; improves thickness and elasticity of vaginal tissues. Caution: Do not use black cohosh in conjunction with estrogen replacement therapy (ERT). Women with estrogen-dependent cancer, including breast, cervical, uterine, and ovarian, should consult their physician before taking it.

Black Cohosh

Chasteberry. Used for smoothing out the hormonal ups and downs of menopause as well as the menstrual cycle and PMS.

Sage. Traditionally used to dry up secretions including perspiration, making it a good choice for helping relieve hot flashes.

St. John's wort. Recognized by the American College of Obstetricians and Gynecologists in Washington, DC, as helpful for treating mild to moderate depression.

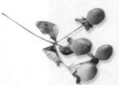

St. John's Wort

Motherwort. Acts on the nervous system to calm heart palpitations caused by menopause.

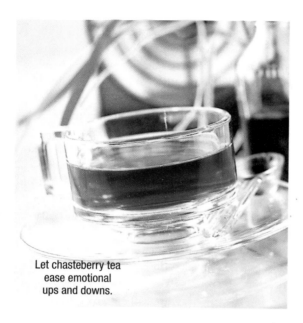

Let chasteberry tea ease emotional ups and downs.

Memory Booster

Hormonal changes can poke holes in your memory and make you feel like you're losing your grip. Disturbed sleep and emotional stress can make matters worse. In my experience, this simple, reliable, and delicious tea, when taken daily for 4 to 6 weeks or so, will help improve your memory. The aroma and flavor are *immediately* invigorating.

½ **tsp dried rosemary**
½ **tsp dried lemon balm**
½ **tsp gotu kola**
½ **tsp ginkgo**

Combine herbs, and steep for 10 minutes in 1 cup boiling water, covered. Strain, and sweeten with honey to taste. Drink 1 to 3 cups daily.

Hot Flash Minimizer

Hot flashes may occur when hormonal changes cause a sudden, temporary spike in body temperature. They can occur at any time, including at night when they're known as night sweats. At night, hot flashes can cause or aggravate insomnia. In time, this symptom will disappear, but you can use the following mixture to minimize hot flashes until they go away for good. You should start to see an improvement within a week or two of taking it regularly.

1 **oz chaste tree tincture**
1 **oz motherwort tincture**
1 **oz hawthorn tincture**
½ **oz black cohosh tincture**
½ **oz sage leaf tincture**

Combine tinctures in a bottle. Take 1 teaspoon in ¼ cup hot water, three times daily.

Mood Booster

Loss of sleep, memory problems, and other physical complaints associated with menopause can fuel depression. For relieving mild depression, try the following formula. Expect to take this for 3 to 6 weeks before you'll feel benefits.

Fruit juice makes tinctures taste better.

Caution: If you are on any medications, check with your doctor or an experienced herbalist before using St. John's wort; it may interfere with their effectiveness. If you are severely depressed or if your mild depression persists past 6 months, consult your health care practitioner. Do not take this formula for longer than 6 months.

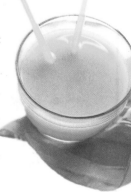

Toss Some Flax on Your Salad

Flaxseed is an excellent source of phytoestrogens (that is, plant estrogens), which may help substitute for some of your naturally declining estrogen. To add flax to your daily diet, simply sprinkle 1 to 2 tablespoons of freshly ground flaxseed onto salads or other foods every day. Or use preground flaxseed: Just be sure to store it in the fridge or freezer. (For you to absorb the benefits of flaxseed, the seeds *must* be ground.)

Like flax, soy products—especially tofu but also tempeh, soybeans, soy milk, soy flour, and soy protein powder—may reduce some risks associated with the drop in estrogen. As a bonus, whole soy foods can help keep cholesterol levels in check and therefore protect your heart. One-half cup tofu or 1 cup soy milk each contains about 30 mg isoflavones, a good amount to aim for each day.

1   oz Siberian ginseng root tincture
1   oz St. John's wort tincture
½   oz vervain tincture
½   oz damiana tincture

Combine these tinctures in a bottle. Take ½ to 1 teaspoon up to four times daily.

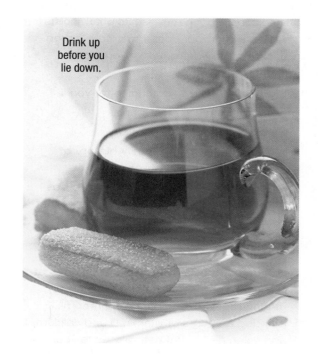

Drink up before you lie down.

‖ Sleep-Enhancing Tea

Night sweats, hormonal rushes, and stress can cause insomnia, which in turn aggravates memory problems. Sip this lovely tea each night an hour before bedtime to help you relax.

1   tsp dried chamomile flowers
1   tsp dried lavender flowers
1   tsp dried lemon balm leaf

Combine herbs, and steep in 1 cup boiling water for 10 minutes, covered. Strain, and sweeten with honey to taste.

An Herbalist's Approach to ERT

Your doctor may recommend that you go on estrogen replacement therapy (ERT), because there's good evidence that these drugs, which maintain your estrogen supply, can help reduce menopausal symptoms and may also protect against osteoporosis and, for some women, heart disease. Today there are a wide variety of ERT formulations on the market. And if you need something fine-tuned for you, your doctor or another licensed medical practitioner can customize a prescription that's filled through a pharmacy that "compounds" (or mixes together) medications upon request. Its pharmacists will work with your doctor to create a product specifically designed for your body chemistry.

ERT may be a good choice for you if

▶ **you have high cholesterol**

▶ **you have low bone density**

▶ **you have a strong family history of heart disease or osteoporosis**

▶ **you're at low risk for some of the possible side effects of ERT such as breast cancer**

If you choose not to use ERT, you can reduce your risks for heart disease and osteoporosis by eating a good, low-fat diet (with plenty of fruits and vegetables), getting regular exercise, taking recommended amounts of vitamin D and calcium, and using herbs that naturally ease your transition to lower estrogen levels, including the herbal remedies mentioned in this chapter.

Insomnia-Relief Tincture

If the Sleep-Enhancing Tea above doesn't help you nod off more easily, try this simple remedy instead. (Caution: This should not be taken with prescription tranquilizers.)

1	oz skullcap tincture
1	oz motherwort tincture
½	oz lavender tincture
½	oz passionflower tincture

Combine tinctures in a bottle, and take ½ teaspoon every 30 minutes for 2 hours before bed. If necessary, take two additional ½-teaspoon doses during the night.

Heart-Calming Tonic

Occasional heart palpitations are common for otherwise healthy, perimenopausal women. Caution: If you notice frequent heart rate or rhythm changes or feel pain, see your doctor promptly, and do not treat yourself with herbs. If you are taking cardiac medications, consult your doctor before taking any herbal remedies, and never adjust your prescribed medications without first consulting your doctor. Use the following formula only for easing heart palpitations associated with menopause. (Note: I also recommend taking 1 teaspoon of this tonic two or three times daily to maintain heart health.)

1	oz motherwort tincture
1	oz lemon balm tincture
1	oz hawthorn tincture
1	oz black cohosh tincture

Combine tinctures in a bottle. For palpitations, take ½ teaspoon every 30 minutes for 2 hours. Relief from palpitations should be evident after one to four doses. Don't take more than 4 teaspoons in any 24-hour period.

CHAPTER 21

Help Your Man Preserve His Potency

Erectile problems are *not* inevitable.
Here's what you—and he—can do

F irst, a statistic that may surprise you: More than half of all men between the ages of 40 and 70 have erectile problems. That translates to an estimated 20 to 30 million men who can't get the erections they want. They're alarming statistics, but don't panic. Thanks to all of the options available today, your man doesn't have to be among them. And if he's suffering from erectile dysfunction (ED) right now, he doesn't have to stay that way. Since

serious health conditions can contribute to erection problems, it's important to make sure the man in your life takes his concerns to his doctor at once. Here are some answers to common questions about ED, and what you and your man can do to keep it out of *your* bedroom.

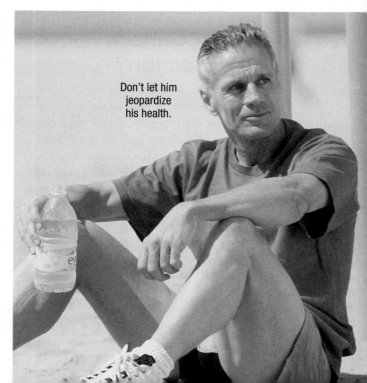

Don't let him
jeopardize
his health.

What Is Erectile Dysfunction?

On any given day (or night), there may be obvious reasons why a man has trouble summoning an erection: stress, fatigue, anxiety, the baby crying in the next room. But if the problem persists, it crosses the line from occasional disappointment to a medical condition called erectile dysfunction (ED). "We usually say that if the problem lasts 3 months or more, you have ED," says Ira Sharlip, MD, spokesperson for the American Urological Association in Baltimore and president of the Sexual Medicine Society of North America in Schaumburg, IL.

The defining symptom of ED is the inability to achieve and maintain an erection sufficient for satisfactory sexual function. While erectile dysfunction is not an uncommon problem among men as they get older, says Dr. Sharlip, neither is it an automatic consequence of aging.

What Causes an Erection?

To know why men sometimes experience equipment failure, you have to understand how erections occur in the first place. Many a man has been accused of thinking with his penis, but in fact the opposite is true: Men have erections with their brains. Whatever the trigger—a romantic evening, a swimsuit catalog—every erection is a sequence of events that begins in his brain, says Tom Lue, MD, professor of urology at the University of California, San Francisco, and spokesperson for the American Foundation for Urologic Disease in Baltimore.

"Basically, when a man is sexually stimulated, a signal is transmitted from the brain down the spinal cord and reaches the penis," he explains. Then the stimulated nerves in the penis release a chemical called a neurotransmitter. This chemical signal causes blood vessels in the penis to open up. Blood is pumped into spongy tissues in the penis, causing it to swell and stiffen, causing an erection.

What Prevents an Erection?

A problem at any step in the erection-making process can cause an erection to be weakened or prevent it altogether. Here are the known erection wreckers.

Low hormone levels. If your man's body isn't producing enough testosterone, the brain-to-penis transmission just won't happen, because he simply won't be aroused. While it's normal for a man's testosterone levels to decrease with age, such changes usually happen gradually and don't completely erase the libido.

Psychological problems. A brain overwhelmed by stress, anxiety, fatigue, or other mental concerns is less likely to send the penis any erection-generating signals.

Don't ignore your man's erection problems. They could be due to life-threatening blockages in his arteries.

Serve Him a Romantic Dessert

"You can awaken a sleepy libido with easy diet changes," contends dietitian Ellen Albertson, coauthor with her chef husband, Michael, of the book *Temptations: Igniting the Pleasure and Power of Aphrodisiacs* (Simon & Schuster, 2002). Besides containing fun recipes using legendary aphrodisiacs from chocolate to chile peppers, this book has tons of practical tips such as these for a better love life.

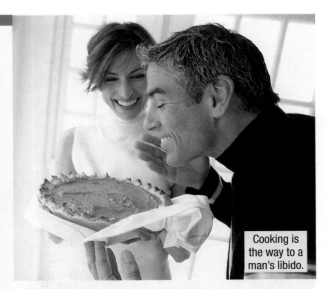

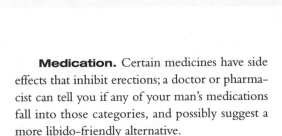

Cooking is the way to a man's libido.

Make him pumpkin pie. Studies in Chicago showed that bloodflow to the penis increased most after men smelled pumpkin pie and lavender. (For women, bloodflow to the vagina increased most from the smells of cucumber and licorice.)

Pour him a cup or two of coffee. An *Archives of Internal Medicine* study showed that coffee drinkers have sex more often and enjoy it more than non–coffee drinkers. A study of older men found that coffee improved sex lives by increasing energy. (Anyone with high blood pressure or migraines should pass on the java.)

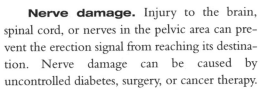

Nerve damage. Injury to the brain, spinal cord, or nerves in the pelvic area can prevent the erection signal from reaching its destination. Nerve damage can be caused by uncontrolled diabetes, surgery, or cancer therapy.

Blocked vessels. If the arteries that bring blood into the erection chamber are blocked, the erection will be weak or even nonexistent.

Damage to the penis. Scar tissue or other structural damage can prevent an erection from occurring.

Medication. Certain medicines have side effects that inhibit erections; a doctor or pharmacist can tell you if any of your man's medications fall into those categories, and possibly suggest a more libido-friendly alternative.

It may seem like there's a lot of things that can go wrong. But low hormone levels, long-term psychological problems, nerve damage, and penis injury are relatively rare causes of ED. The problem that most men should be concerned about is blocked arteries. "High blood pressure, high cholesterol, coronary artery disease: People with these conditions will also have trouble pumping blood into the penis," says Dr. Lue. It's the same process that leads to heart disease: Arteries become gunked up, and the narrowed channels can't bring in enough blood to do the job.

In a study of 50 men experiencing impotence, 40% had significant blockages in their coronary arteries, though they had no other symptoms of vascular disease. That makes ED an early warning signal of heart disease and stroke.

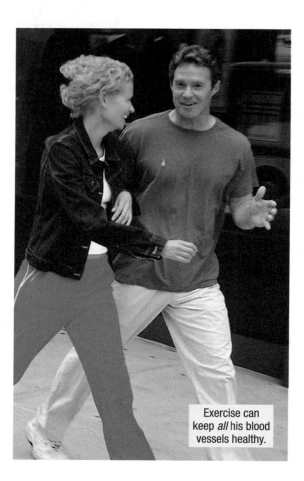

Exercise can keep *all* his blood vessels healthy.

What Can the Doctor Do to Help?

When you and your husband talk to his family doctor about his erection problems, odds are he'll write a prescription for sildenafil citrate, known as Viagra. "It works for two-thirds of the men who try it," Dr. Sharlip says. "It's the first-line treatment for ED."

Viagra does its job by causing the chemical messenger that stimulates erections to persist in your man's body longer than it normally would. This keeps narrowed blood vessels open, allowing an erection to occur. This medicine doesn't produce erections; rather, it sets the stage for them to occur naturally. "A man still needs some sort of sexual stimulation for an erection to happen," says Dr. Lue. His doctor will typically instruct him to take Viagra 1 hour before sex.

Warning: For some men, particularly those with serious heart conditions or those taking certain other medicines, particularly any drug containing nitrate (notable nitroglycerin), Viagra can be deadly. Make sure your man tells his doctor what drugs he's taking before accepting *any* new medication, especially Viagra.

If Viagra doesn't work (or isn't an option) for your man, his doctor will refer him to a urologist who will do a more specialized examination. Depending on the cause of his erectile dysfunction, there are a number of other options for treatment, including injections, capsules, a vacuum device, surgery, or even an implant.

The bottom line: "A man who's willing to do whatever is necessary has a 90 to 95% chance of having satisfactory sexual functioning for the rest of his life," says Dr. Sharlip.

1-MINUTE *HEALTH BOOSTER*

Consider a Sex Therapist

If this sounds too racy for you, let us put your mind at ease. The sexy stuff is actually done at home with your partner, not during the office visits. "In a typical session, the therapist will ask the couple a series of detailed questions about what's happening or not happening. Then he'll give them behavior-oriented homework assignments," explains Gerald Weeks, PhD, chairman of the department of counseling at the University of Nevada–Las Vegas and author of several textbooks for doctors and sex therapists.

Sex therapists, especially those who also do marital therapy, can make medical treatments more effective by helping couples deal with psychological issues that may be contributing to erectile dysfunction (ED). They can also help couples get their sex lives back on track after a long dry spell and advise them on how to bring various medical therapies into the bedroom.

Sex therapy doesn't mean signing up for years of analysis; most problems can be overcome in a matter of 10 to 15 one-hour sessions, says Dr. Weeks. To find a board-certified sex therapist, visit the Web sites of the American Board of Sexology (www.sexologist.org) and the American Association of Sex Educators, Counselors, and Therapists (www.aasect.org).

What Can You Do to Help?

If you want your man's ability to have erections to stick around for the next few decades, he'll need to implement a few erection-friendly lifestyle changes starting today. Here's what doctors say is necessary.

Help him quit smoking. Amazingly, there are still men for whom the threat of an early death isn't motivation enough to quit. So how about the threat of an early death after years without sex? Smoking is as bad for the arteries that support an erection as it is for the arteries that nourish his heart.

Encourage him to eat healthier. A healthy diet will help him lose weight and lower his cholesterol, keeping him alive longer and, very possibly, keeping him erect longer. Just feed him the meals you're eating thanks to Chapter 2!

Get him to exercise with you. Exercise will help him shed pounds, lower his blood pressure, and keep his blood vessels healthy, including those critical ones in the groin area.

Have sex regularly. Besides making you both feel good and strengthening your relationship, having and using his erections may help keep his penis in working order. Which, of course, allows him to keep having and using erections in the future.

Your Yearly Exam Planner

Use this handy worksheet to help give your gynecologist a more accurate update

Every time you go in for your yearly exam, the gynecologist asks when the first day of your last period was, and you always give an answer. But be honest: Do you usually *know* the answer or do you just give an educated guess? Telling even *little* fibs to your doctor means that she's not getting the clearest possible picture of your reproductive and sexual health. That's why we came up with this handy worksheet for you to fill out and take to the doctor's the next time you have your annual checkup. Be as specific as you can with dates and diagnoses. And use the space below to record any questions you have so you'll remember to ask them!

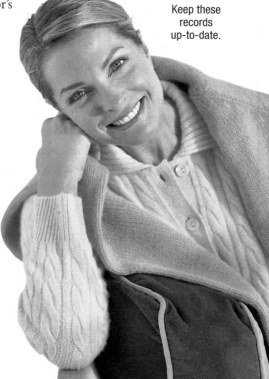

Keep these records up-to-date.

Questions I have:

Name: _____ Date of Birth: _____

Reproductive History

▶ Age at which you first got your period _____
▶ Contraceptive use _____
▶ Breast health (cysts, surgery, cancer, etc.) _____
▶ Sexually transmitted diseases _____
▶ Number of pregnancies _____
▶ Difficulties during or after pregnancies _____
▶ Miscarriages, stillbirths, childhood deaths, abortions_____
▶ Depression (postpartum or otherwise)_____

Family Reproductive History

▶ Breast cancer_____
▶ Other reproductive cancers _____
▶ Colon cancer_____
▶ Thyroid or other hormonal conditions _____
▶ Age at which your mother entered menopause _____
▶ Heart disease _____
▶ Osteoporosis _____
▶ Depression (postpartum or otherwise) _____

Test Result Information

▶ Abnormal Pap test results _____
▶ Abnormal mammogram results _____
▶ Abnormal biopsy results _____

Recent Personal History

(to be filled out just prior to your exam)

▶ Start and end dates of your most recent period _____
▶ Changes in menstruation*_____
▶ Lumps noticed during breast self-exams*_____
▶ Breast discomfort _____
▶ Pelvic floor problems (see p. 134) _____
▶ Urinary tract infections or urine leakage _____
▶ Sexual problems or discomfort _____
▶ Birth control questions or concerns _____
▶ Additional questions _____

If you feel any lumps or notice any other changes in your breasts or in your menstrual cycle, especially if the change involves additional bleeding, call your gynecologist immediately. Also call your doctor if you experience a dramatic change in volume of menstrual flow more for than one cycle (such as going from using three pads a day to four or five).

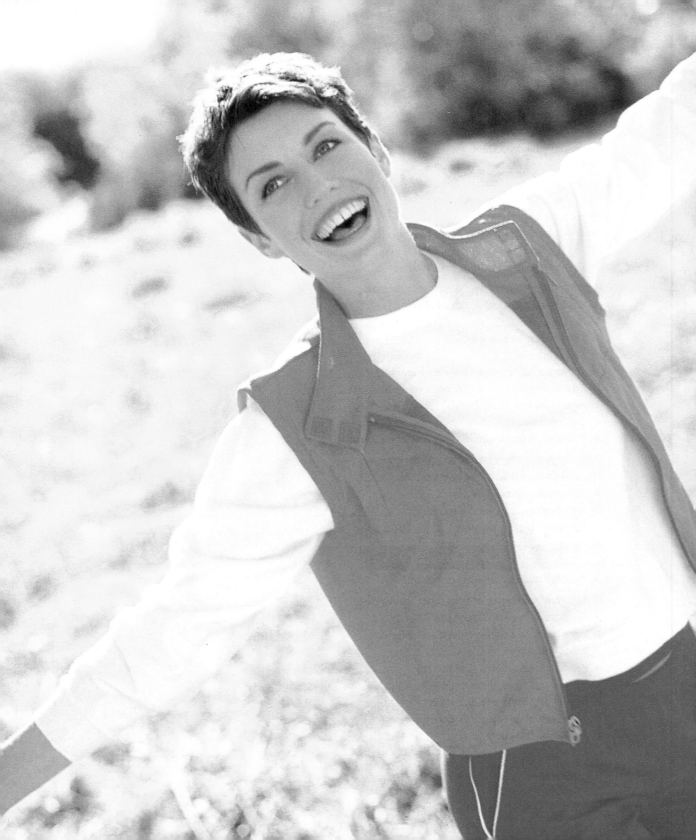

Everyday Health Boosters

CHAPTER 22

Double Your Energy!

These easy tips will help you get revved up and feel fantastic—right now!

In our 24/7 world, 40 million Americans suffer from sleep disorders, and more than half of all adults report feeling high stress every day. So if you find yourself feeling like your battery's been drained, you're certainly not alone.

Fortunately, there are plenty of simple ways to boost your energy every day: breathing more deeply, sitting up straighter, having a few good belly laughs, and getting a little extra sunlight and exercise, to name just a few.

Here's how these and the four other natural energy-enhancers in this chapter work. Replace your usual coffee breaks with the following healthy habits, and you'll be ready to take on the world with energy to spare!

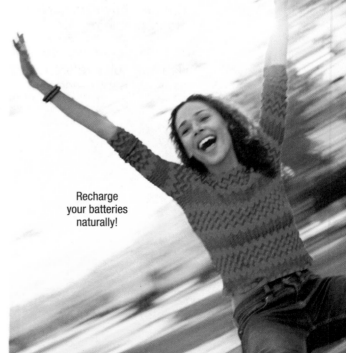

Recharge
your batteries
naturally!

Invigorate Your Body with Belly Breathing

"People are so overwhelmed by everything they think they must do that they rarely take time to just breathe," says Monica Myklebust, MD, a family physician in the Program in Integrative Medicine at the University of Arizona in Tucson. "Proper breathing helps quiet body and mind, which can shift our perspective and refresh the spirit."

Yet many people in Western society don't breathe correctly, she says. Taught to suck in our guts and puff out our chests, we're a nation of shallow "chest breathers." Few people—other than musicians and some athletes—are even aware that the abdomen should expand during inhalation to allow maximum expansion of the lungs.

Taking a deep belly breath is a surefire way to invigorate body and mind anytime throughout the day, says Dr. Myklebust.

How to do it: Sit in a comfortable chair with your legs uncrossed and your spine tall. Breathe in slowly through your nose so that the air completely fills your lungs down into your belly, expanding your abdomen. Breathe out slowly through your nose. Inhale to the count of three (1, 2, 3), then exhale to the count of two (4, 5). Breathe in smooth cycles without pausing. Start with 2 minutes of breathwork, and work up to 5 to 10 minutes, with 12 breath cycles per minute. If desired, focus on a candle, flower, or meaningful picture, or play music to enhance your practice.

1-MINUTE HEALTH BOOSTER

Energize Your Workout Instantly!

Dragging in the gym? Dab some peppermint oil on your collar. In a study at Wheeling Jesuit University in West Virginia, 40 athletes ran faster and did more push-ups when exposed to peppermint scent than those with other or no scents. "Peppermint boosts mood," explains researcher Bryan Raudenbush, PhD, "so you perform better without working harder."

Minty breath may boost stamina.

Seek Energy-Boosting Sunlight

"One reason for the fatigue that is rampant in our society may be light deprivation," explains Michael Terman, PhD, director of clinical chronobiology at the New York State Psychiatric Institute in New York City. Research suggests that exposure to artificial bright light therapy in the early morning can boost energy throughout the day, notes Dr. Terman.

Walking, jogging, or doing any form of exercise in sunlight boosts this energy-enhancing power, he says. While exposure to sunlight any-

Something as simple as taking deeper breaths can have a profound impact on your energy level.

time can provide a pick me-up, Dr. Terman explains that "the dawn signal has a particularly strong therapeutic effect."

How to do it: Take a walk outdoors for 30 to 45 minutes every day, preferably right after you wake up. Even a cloudy day offers enough light photons to have a stimulating effect on the brain.

Prepare Your Body for Motion

"People think good posture is about doing something, such as tightening the abdominals, but it's actually more about being ready to move," says Andrea Wiener, assistant director of the Feldenkrais Guild of North America in Portland,

How Exercise Fires You Up

If you think your lack of energy is because you don't get enough sleep or have too much to do, you may be pinning your fatigue on the wrong bad habit. Surprisingly, few people recognize that one of the main reasons for their personal energy crisis is the lack of exercise, says James S. Gordon, MD, director of the Center for Mind-Body Medicine in Washington, DC, and chairman of the White House Commission on Complementary and Alternative Medicine Policy.

"Everyone's always rushing, often under great pressure, so they feel like they're doing a lot," says Dr. Gordon, who prescribes a daily dose of physical activity for all his patients. "But in fact, we live in an extremely sedentary society. Most people get very little physical activity and hold a tremendous amount of tension in their body—all of which is exhausting." Although it may seem contradictory, expending energy can actually *increase* your energy. Here's how:

It relieves tension and keeps you alert. Walking, stretching, and other forms of movement help relieve muscle tension and send oxygenated blood to the brain and other vital organs.

It builds stamina. Regular exercise boosts the efficiency of the heart and lungs, making the tasks of daily life easier and less tiring.

It keeps you slim. Physically active people are less likely to gain excess pounds that can literally weigh them down.

It helps you sleep. Studies show that fit people sleep better, fall asleep quicker, wake up less often, and experience more delta sleep—the deepest sleep of the night, which promotes the greatest amount of body recovery.

It keeps you healthy. Regular physical activity can help prevent and relieve a host of energy-draining ailments, from the common cold to certain cancers.

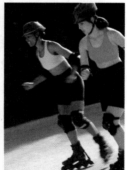

Move your body to boost your mood.

It improves mood. Exercise rids the body of stress hormones, brightening mood and relieving feelings of depression and anxiety.

OR, which teaches people healthy movement habits. Just as an Olympic athlete balances effort and relaxation so that all motion goes toward results, good standing posture relies on muscles to let your skeleton support your body, Wiener says.

How to do it: Stand in your normal posture. Now prepare to jump up, and notice how your posture changes. Prepare to jump forward, then backward, then to the right and the left. Pay attention to your posture change for each movement. Posture that allows you to move instantly in any direction is good posture. To learn more about the Feldenkrais method, call (800) 775-2118, or go to the Web site at www.feldenkrais.com.

Stretch Away Desk Fatigue

America's epidemic of neck, shoulder, and back pain results from being "a nation of slouchers," says Hope Gillerman, spokeswoman for the American Society for the Alexander Technique in Florence, MA. This technique is a form of movement therapy that helps people relieve pain by correcting their body's alignment.

Hunched over steering wheels and computer keyboards, people can easily develop a round-shouldered posture that forces them to tighten muscles to support the head, which weighs 10 to 15 lb. Gillerman notes that "most people are locked into habitual patterns of tension and strain that cause them to use much more force and energy than necessary." Try the following exercise, based on a lesson of the Alexander Technique.

How to do it: Sit on the front edge of a chair with both feet flat on the floor and your body weight evenly distributed on your two

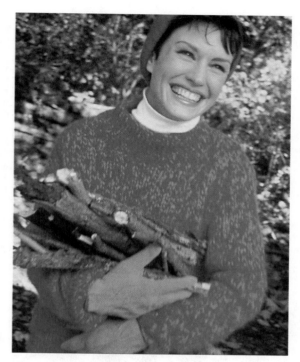

Staying active throughout the day will help keep you going strong from dawn till dusk.

pelvic sitting bones. Clasp your hands with fingers interlocked, and lift your arms overhead, palms to the ceiling. Stretch your spine up while keeping your gaze forward. Release your hands as you relax your arms down by your sides, keeping the spine lengthened. Then, exhale completely, inhale gently, and exhale again as you relax the muscles of your shoulders, arms, neck, face, and back.

For information on the Alexander Technique, call (800) 473-0620; in Canada, call (416) 631-8127; or go online to their Web site at www.alexandertech.org.

Burn Calories, Boost Energy

"Physical fitness is the cornerstone of energy," contends Connie Tyne, executive director of The Cooper Wellness Program in Dallas, a sort of summer camp for grown-ups where participants learn how to integrate healthy habits into their life. "The fitter you are, the less work it takes to do any task," says Tyne.

You don't have to join a gym or spend lots of time to get fit, she says. Studies from The Cooper Institute for Research show that everyday "lifestyle activities" (such as taking the stairs and parking in the farthest space) can provide health benefits similar to a traditional gym workout. What's more, these "fit bits" offer an immediate energy boost by pumping oxygenated blood through the body.

How to do it: "Look for simple ways to add movement into your life," advises Tyne, who gets in a strength training workout each night by doing calisthenics such as sit-ups and push-ups for 10 minutes while watching the news.

Here are other easy ways to energize and get fit, bit by bit: Stand up and stretch when your computer is downloading or printing, move around while you're talking on a cordless phone, and walk your dog twice a day.

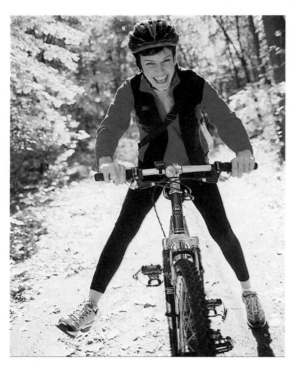

Get playful! Laughter actually has both energizing and healing powers!

Liven Up with a Laugh

"Laughter is like internal jogging," wrote author Norman Cousins in his classic book, *Anatomy of an Illness*. Cousins used humor to help heal himself from a debilitating disease. He found that 10 minutes of belly laughter (brought on by watching comedies such as *Candid Camera*) gave him 2 hours of pain-free sleep.

Scientific evidence now supports laughter's healing and energizing power, according to Joel Goodman, director of The Humor Project, Inc., in Saratoga Springs, NY. "A good laugh has many positive physiologic effects," he contends, "such as boosting immune function, enhancing respiration, and lowering levels of stress hormones."

How to do it: Create a "mirth aid kit" with books, videos, and funny props, so you can

DO JUST ONE THING!

Get Your Iron Levels Checked

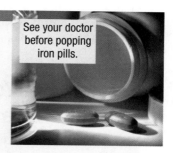

See your doctor before popping iron pills.

Iron is a key part of hemoglobin, the protein in red blood cells that carries oxygen throughout your body, and a deficiency in this mineral can leave you dragging. It's also the most common deficiency in the US, with about 15% of American women at risk of iron deficiency anemia, says Sean Lynch, MD, of Eastern Virginia Medical School in Norfolk. Premenopausal women who lose iron during menstruation are the most likely candidates, particularly if they don't eat meat. Iron deficiency is especially bad news in pregnant women, because it can boost the risk of delivering premature and low birth-weight babies. Still, iron supplements are nothing to be taken lightly; too much iron can be harmful. Here's what you need to know:

If you're run-down, don't buy iron supplements unless your doctor advises you to do so. Too much iron can be dangerous, particularly for people with certain genetic conditions. Instead, see your doctor for a blood test to check for both anemia and low iron stores, also known as ferritin levels, recommends John Beard, PhD, professor of nutrition at Pennsylvania State University in State College. If you have low ferritin levels, it won't take much (an illness, pregnancy, surgery) to deplete your reserves and leave you anemic.

If your doctor finds that you do have anemia or low ferritin levels, he'll probably prescribe iron supplements. How much and for how long depends on how severe the problem is, says Dr. Lynch.

The iron in supplements is best absorbed on an empty stomach. Try taking iron supplements a few hours after you've eaten, particularly if you've had coffee, tea, or foods high in bran, soy protein, or calcium, all of which further lessen iron absorption.

If iron supplements make you nauseous, take them with a vitamin C-rich food or drink. While food decreases iron absorption, C boosts the absorption of supplemental iron. If this doesn't help, ask your doctor about chelated iron or time-release iron supplements, Dr. Lynch advises.

To prevent iron deficiency anemia, eat lean beef, legumes, fortified cereals, and other iron-rich foods. Premenopausal women should also take a multi containing 100% of the Daily Value for iron. Deficiency is uncommon in postmenopausal women (or in men over 18), so there's little reason to take extra iron if you fall into this group (unless your doctor advises you to do so).

take a dose of hilarity whenever you need it. For more ideas, visit www.humorproject.com.

Refresh Yourself with Yoga

Yoga stretches can wake up a tired body, especially if you've been sitting too long, says Sara Ivanhoe, a Santa Monica, CA, yoga instructor, star of the video *Yoga for Dummies*, and president

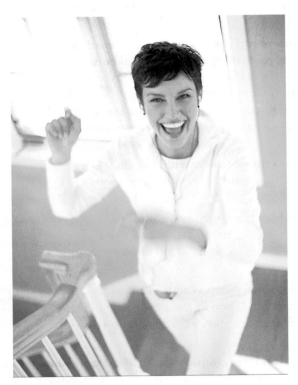

For an energy boost anytime, crank up the tunes, and dance away the blues!

of yoganation.com. "Poses that open the chest, such as back bends, are especially invigorating, because they expand breathing capacity and stimulate the nervous system. And some inversions, in which the head is lower than the heart, boost energy by sending blood to the brain."

How to do it: An easy yoga chest opener and gentle inversion is the "puppy dog," a modification of the classic "downward facing dog." Stand facing a wall, and place your hands against the wall at about hip height. Walk backward until your back is parallel to the floor, and your body creates a sort of box with the walls and floor. Relax your head, and press your palms into the wall with your fingers spread wide and your middle finger pointing toward the ceiling. Soften your knees, and extend your tailbone up. Take a few deep breaths as you focus on lengthening your spine, then release. For more great yoga stretches, turn to Chapter 10.

Dance Away from Stress

When people say they're too tired to exercise, their fatigue is often emotional rather than physical, says Rebecca Gorrell, a movement therapist at Canyon Ranch Health Resort in Tucson. "Movement can help people shift their energy, stabilize their emotions, and bring a profound sense of joy," she explains. "But we need to forget the Western, military approach to exercise, which is all about harder, faster, higher." Instead, adopt a more Eastern view of "mindful exercise," picking any form of movement you enjoy and find nourishing. "For many people, this is dance," Gorrell says. "Almost every culture dances as part of ritual and art, so it's almost encoded in our DNA."

How to do it: Play music you like, Gorrell suggests, moving your body to the rhythm in whatever way it needs. For example, if you're angry, you may want to stomp around and punch pillows. If you're sad, you may want to sway. Expressing emotions through your body can relieve and refresh your mind.

Rest and Relax— with Intensity!

"Too often when we're tired, we reach for something—such as food or coffee—to cover it up," says Judith Hanson Lasater, PhD, a San Francisco physical therapist and yoga instructor who holds a doctorate in East-West psychology. "But what we really need at times like that is to give in to the fatigue so we can release it."

Taking as little as 5 to 10 minutes "to do a period of intense nothing" or deep relaxation can be tremendously restorative, says Dr. Lasater, who presents varied yoga postures that encourage deep rest in her book *Relax and Renew* (Rodmell Press, 1995). For more information, visit www.judithlasater.com.

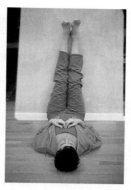

This comfortable pose will relax you and restore and renew your energy.

How to do it: One of Dr. Lasater's simplest strategies is to set a timer; then give yourself permission to "stop doing and just be" until the timer goes off.

Lie on your back—with your legs resting up on a wall if you'd like—and relax all of your muscles, letting the weight of your body melt into the floor. Take deep abdominal breaths, and totally give yourself over to the experience of letting go.

CHAPTER 23

Defeat Germs *Before* They Make You Sick

These herbs prevent and treat sinusitis, yeast infections, bronchitis, acne, and more!

W hether it's "cold season" or not, your immune system is constantly under assault from infections. Its job: to get bacteria, viruses, fungi, and cancer cells—before they get you. But in order for your immune system to do its job, you've got to keep it healthy. You must eat right, sleep right, exercise regularly, and keep stress to a minimum. In short: *Take care of yourself.*

Beyond that, you can help give your immune system an extra edge when it comes to preventing and fighting infection by jump-starting it with some of Mother Nature's own immunity-boosting herbs. In this chapter, you'll find three of the best, along with tips on when to use them and how much to take—all straight from *Prevention*'s own herb expert

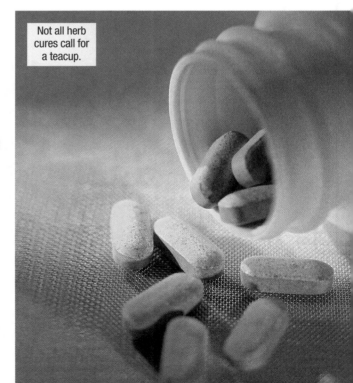

Not all herb cures call for a teacup.

Douglas Schar, DipPhyt, MCPP, MNIMH, a European-trained clinical herbalist with practices in London and Washington, DC.

A word of caution before we get to the herbs: Some infections—including Lyme disease, staph, and others—can be deadly if they're not treated with antibiotics or other prescription medications. So be sure to call your physician the moment you suspect you've got something serious. See "When to See the Doctor" at right for some important guidelines.

‖ The Bacteria Beater

Echinacea
(Echinacea angustifolia)

Used by Native Americans to heal skin injuries, echinacea was applied topically and taken internally to keep bites, wounds, and burns infection-free. Physicians later learned that when patients took echinacea, their immune-cell counts skyrocketed. Numerous studies have confirmed this action. Keep a bottle on hand in your medicine chest at all times.

When to Take Echinacea

To fight bacterial and viral infections. Take it when symptoms emerge and for 2 weeks after you begin to feel better.

To treat chronic infections. If you've been diagnosed with recurrent urinary tract infections (bacterial cystitis, urethritis), respiratory infections (sinusitis, bronchitis, tonsillitis), or skin infections (erysipelas), use echinacea for 3 months to break the cycle.

For acne (chronic or cyclical). For chronic acne, try using echinacea for 3 months. If the condition clears, continue taking it for an additional 3 months. If the problem is cyclical, try

When to See the Doctor

Above all, use common sense. If you're worried about an infection, call the doctor right away or go to the emergency room, if necessary. Here are other indications that a doctor visit is in order:

▶ **Your infection is not responding.**

▶ **Your symptoms are getting worse (especially if they deteriorate rapidly).**

▶ **Your fever spikes or persists for more than 48 hours.**

▶ **An infected wound is red, hot, and full of pus.**

▶ **A urinary tract infection is accompanied by a high fever and back pain. (In this case, see a doctor *immediately*.)**

using echinacea the minute you sense an outbreak is on its way, then continue using it for 2 weeks.

For earaches. Ear infections are tough to treat because ears have poor circulation, which means that the antibiotics you take to cure an earache have a hard time getting where they need to go. Use echinacea at the first sign of an earache, and continue using it for 2 weeks after the pain disappears.

For wounds. When you get a scratch, minor cut, insect bite, or burn, the "seal" on the body breaks, giving bacteria an easy entry point into your body. An immune stimulant—used both internally and externally—can keep minor wounds infection-free. Spray echinacea tincture onto the wound three times a day while also tak-

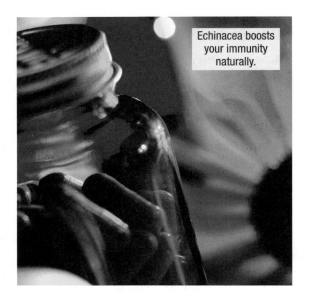

Echinacea boosts your immunity naturally.

How to Use Echinacea

Only buy products made from echinacea root. Avoid all products made with leaves. Avoid "standardized" products.

> **Dosage:** Take one dose three times a day.
> ▶ **Tableted dried root:** two 500-mg tablets
> ▶ **Echinacea root tincture 1:5:** 1 teaspoon (5 ml)
> ▶ **Echinacea root tincture 1:1:** 20 drops

The Fungus and Virus Vanquisher

Maitake (*Grifola frondosa*)

The Romans and ancient Japanese coveted this mushroom as a delicacy. More recently, researchers have found that maitake inhibits the spread of cancer. Intrigued, they probed the mushroom for cancer-killing compounds, but found none. Further research showed that rather than attacking cancer cells directly, maitake stimulates the immune system to kill them.

Completely nontoxic, maitake is an excellent option for viral infections too. The viruses that cause coughs, colds, influenza, warts, herpes, and chronic fatigue syndrome are all given a run for

ing echinacea internally until the wound has entirely healed, and the scab has fallen off.

Before a hospital visit. Hospitals are breeding grounds for really nasty bacteria. If you're going to the hospital—for a visit or a stay—use echinacea to keep your immune system fired up. If possible, take it a week before a hospital visit and for a week following the visit. If it's a spur-of-the-moment visit, take echinacea for a week following the visit.

Give Infections a One-Two Punch

"I often advise people who are taking antibiotics to also take an herbal immune enhancer," says Douglas Schar, DipPhyt, MCPP, MNIMH, a European-trained clinical herbalist with practices in London and Washington, DC. "These herbs work on a different and unrelated level and are therefore safe to use at the same time. Antibiotics kill bugs. Herbal immune enhancers stimulate the immune system to kill bugs. I think it's a winning double whammy, especially for fighting bacterial infection."

their money with this herb. Maitake is also tops when it comes to eradicating fungal infections such as yeast infections, athlete's foot, and jock itch.

When to Take Maitake

To prevent illness (as in, you've been exposed to something and are afraid you'll catch it). Say the kids brought a virus home from school, or a nasty cold is whipping through the office. Take maitake for 2 weeks following exposure.

To lessen the severity of coughs and colds. Antibiotics attack only bacteria; they do nothing for these viral conditions. Use maitake to keep coughs and colds under control. Take it while the cough or cold is raging and for 2 weeks beyond the point when you feel well.

To stay healthy on vacation. Getting a cold while on vacation is an unpleasant—yet common—phenomenon. It's stressful getting out the door and on the road, and this depresses immunity. When we take our depressed immunity onto trains, planes, and boats and expose it to hundreds of people and all their bugs, trouble

often occurs. To avoid this, use maitake for 1 week before you go on vacation, for the duration of the trip, and for 1 week after you get home.

How to Use Maitake

Only buy products containing dried maitake. Avoid those that contain other herbs.

> **Dosage:** Take one dose three times a day.
> ▶ **Infection prevention:** two 350-mg tablets
> ▶ **During an infection:** four 350-mg tablets

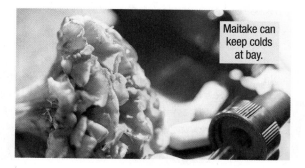
Maitake can keep colds at bay.

Boost Immunity with Instant Workouts

Studies have shown that doing two or three short exercise sessions throughout the day can give you the same fitness benefits as one long bout. Now researchers at Texas Christian University in Fort Worth think they've found another important benefit to multiple workouts: a boost in immunity.

In a small study, 10 volunteers rode a stationary bike for 60 minutes in the morning and again in the afternoon, while another group remained sedentary. One week later, the subjects switched places and repeated the experiment. The researchers found that not only did the exercisers have significantly higher counts of important immune system cells than the nonexercisers, but their immunity was even higher after the *second* bout of exercise.

Fortunately, you don't have to pedal 2 hours a day to benefit, according to lead researcher Brian McFarlin, LAT (licensed athletic trainer), a PhD candidate in exercise physiology at Purdue University in West Lafayette, IN. "Though we need more research to understand the exercise/immunity connection, the benefit seems to come from multiple bouts of activity, which is great news for busy people. When you can't find a 30- or 45-minute block of time to exercise, your immunity may benefit even more by grabbing a few shorter workouts throughout the day," says McFarlin.

The Resistance Builder

Astragalus
(Astragalus membranaceus)

An Asian plant, astragalus is a traditional Chinese vitality tonic used to remedy weakness, fatigue, senility, and that general run-down feeling. Contemporary researchers have found it to be a first-class immune stimulant that increases immune cell counts and activity. Some experts recommend it for people who are worn out and fatigued. Indeed, studies indicate that astragalus even increases immune function for people undergoing chemotherapy and radiation therapy for cancer. No get up and go? Go and get some astragalus!

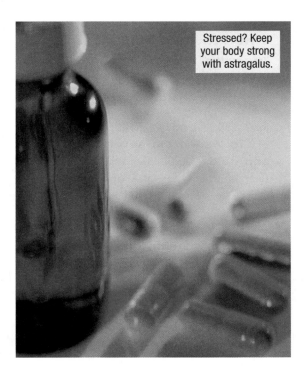

Stressed? Keep your body strong with astragalus.

When to Take Astragalus

To nip infection in the bud. You can just feel it when a cold's on the way: You're tired, achy, and irritable, and all you want to do is nap. Start taking astragalus when you feel the first signs of an infection, and continue taking it for 2 weeks.

To boost resistance during those stressful periods. Whether it's an insanely tight work deadline or a bad patch in your personal life, stress leaves your body vulnerable to infection. Use astragalus to fire up your immune system when you know your resistance is being weakened by stress. It's bad enough to be under stress, but even worse to be under stress *and* sick. Use astragalus during your period of stress and for 2 weeks after the stress has subsided.

To counter age-related lowered immunity. Call it another design flaw of the human body: As we get older, our immune function declines. But you don't have to take this situation lying down. People over the age of 60 may want to take astragalus during the cold and flu season and for 2 months in the summer to get their immune systems out of retirement and back on active duty.

How to Use Astragalus

Avoid products that contain other herbs.

Dosage: Take one dose three times a day:
- ▶ **Tableted dried root:** two 500-mg tablets
- ▶ **Tincture 1:5:** 1 teaspoon (5 ml)
- ▶ **Tincture 1:1:** 20 drops

CHAPTER **24**

Get a Good Night's Sleep—Finally

How one woman found relief from a common sleep disorder, and how you can too!

In this chapter, we bring you a unique success story: A first-person account of a woman who spent every day hovering at the brink of exhaustion. She, like most people, would dream, roll over, and talk in her sleep. She went to bed every night at 10:00 PM and slept until 6:45 AM. She thought that she was getting a typical night's rest, so she couldn't understand why, when the alarm went off in the morning, she was so tired that she'd find herself planning her afternoon nap while she was making the bed.

Thanks to finally being diagnosed with—and treated for—a common sleep disorder, this story has a happy ending. Today, the very same woman (who prefers to remain anonymous) enjoys peaceful, restful sleep. Her hope? That in telling her story, she can help other women do the same.

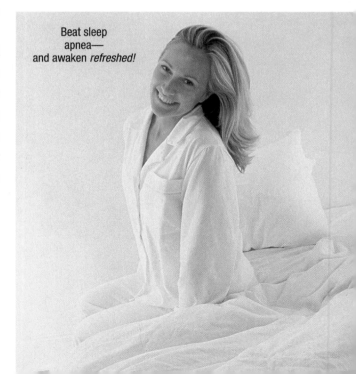

Beat sleep apnea— and awaken *refreshed!*

The Problem Emerges

My problem came on so gradually that I hardly noticed any changes at all. For as long as I could remember, I have felt chronically sleep deprived. I felt tired all the time and had no energy to do the work I needed to do. I would work as hard as I could in the mornings, knowing that by 1:00 in the afternoon, I would become saddled with what experts call excessive daytime sleepiness, or EDS. Once the afternoon rolled around, I wouldn't be able to keep my eyes open and would feel compelled to take a nap.

And I'm not just talking a 15-minute catnap either. (How I envied people who could feel alive again after just 15 minutes!) My naps would last 3 to 4 hours, and I would still awaken unrefreshed, usually feeling worse than when I lay down. I was depressed, because I thought I just couldn't cope as well as everyone else. And I didn't know how much longer I could keep functioning this way.

As it turned out, the solution to my problem came from my husband: He'd been complaining of my snoring for years; in fact, he wore earplugs to bed every night and, even then, often had to go into self-exile on the downstairs couch to get away from the din. Then one morning, pretty much out of the blue, he suggested that I see our family doctor to find out whether I might have sleep apnea.

What Is Sleep Apnea?

Apnea is a Greek word that means "without breath." The sleep disorder that bears the name

---

1-MINUTE *HEALTH BOOSTER*

Check Your "Snore Score"

Your answers to this quiz will help you figure out whether you suffer from sleep apnea.

1. Do you snore loudly and often?

Yes ❏   No ❏

2. Do you feel tired and groggy when you wake up? Yes ❏   No ❏

3. Are you often sleepy during waking hours? Yes ❏   No ❏

4. Are you overweight and/or have a thick neck? Yes ❏   No ❏

5. Has someone told you that you choke, gasp, or hold your breath while you sleep? Yes ❏   No ❏

If you or someone close to you answered yes to any of the above questions, discuss your symptoms with your physician or a sleep specialist.

Quiz courtesy of the American Sleep Apnea Association

---

is as common as adult diabetes, affecting as many as 18 million Americans. Some experts believe that upward of 90% of the cases remain undiagnosed.

Although I had heard about this sleep disorder before, I assumed that only overweight men age 40 and older were susceptible to it. The truth is that sleep apnea can hit anyone: men, women, children, and people of normal weight. And it tends to run in families. For example, I'm a normal-weight female in my early 40s, but my father, sister, and brother all snore. In fact, my sister and brother have sleep studies scheduled to put an end to *their* daytime sleepiness.

There are three types of sleep apnea: obstructive, central, and mixed. The most common, obstructive sleep apnea, occurs when soft tissue in the back of the throat collapses and obstructs the airway, causing you to repeatedly stop breathing during sleep. With central sleep apnea, the brain doesn't signal your muscles to breathe, although your airway isn't blocked.

Mixed sleep apnea is a combination of obstructive and central. Two of the most common symptoms of apnea, particularly the obstructive and mixed types, are excessive daytime sleepiness (falling asleep easily and sometimes inappropriately) and loud snoring.

The Sleep Apnea Pattern

Here's what happens: When you fall asleep, the muscles that stiffen the airway behind the tongue and soft palate relax. If the airway is normal in size, this poses no problems. However, if the airway is small (excess weight is the most common culprit, and genetics is the other), it can close shut. Breathing continues against the closed airway and becomes increasingly vigorous as blood oxygen levels drop and carbon dioxide levels increase. The increasing effort to breathe eventually causes you to arouse or briefly awaken, which activates the muscles, reopening the airway. Because the arousals are brief, and you return to

DO JUST ONE THING!

Log On for More Info

For more information about sleep apnea (for yourself or someone else), contact any of the following organizations. For a link to certified sleep centers near you, go to www.aasmnet.org/search2.htm.

American Academy of Sleep Medicine
6301 Bandel Rd. NW, Suite 101
Rochester, MN 55901
www.aasmnet.org
(507) 287-6006

American Sleep Apnea Association
1424 K St. NW, Suite 302
Washington, DC 20005
www.sleepapnea.org
(202) 293-3650

National Center on Sleep Disorders Research
Two Rockledge Centre
6701 Rockledge Dr., Suite 10038
Bethesda, MD 20892
www.nhlbi.nih.gov/health/public/sleep
(301) 435-0199

National Sleep Foundation
1522 K Street NW, Suite 500
Washington, DC 20005
www.sleepfoundation.org
(202) 347-3471

sleep quickly, you are unaware that they are occurring. If this process recurs frequently during the night, sleep becomes fragmented and non-restorative, and daytime sleepiness or fatigue results.

Not only can sleep apnea rob you of your joie de vivre, but it can be dangerous. In fact, a recent Canadian study showed that if left untreated, obstructive sleep apnea makes a person three times more likely to be involved in a motor vehicle accident than people without the disorder. Untreated sleep apnea can also affect your ability to concentrate, can cause memory problems, weight gain, and feelings of depression, and may contribute to cardiovascular disease, high blood pressure, and stroke.

Getting Answers

When my husband brought up the possibility that I might have sleep apnea, I was actually a little relieved. If I could just find out what was wrong, I could do something about my unrelenting fatigue. So I made an appointment with my internist. After asking me questions about my snoring and daytime sleepiness and hearing my textbook sleep apnea answers, he referred me to a sleep specialist for a consultation.

My appointment was with pulmonologist Richard Strobel, MD, director of the Lehigh Valley Hospital Sleep Disorders Center in Allentown, PA. He peered down my throat and into my ears, then reviewed a questionnaire I had filled out about my sleep, nap, and lifestyle habits. Because he wasn't certain that I had sleep apnea, he suggested that I have a sleep study to find out.

Mine would be a split-night sleep study: For the first half of the night, polysomnographic tech-

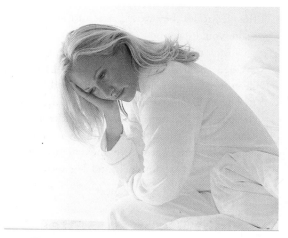

Two common symptoms of sleep apnea: excessive daytime sleepiness and loud snoring.

nologists (people specially trained to administer sleep studies) would monitor how I slept without a Continuous Positive Airway Pressure, or CPAP (pronounced see-pap), machine. CPAP therapy, the most effective treatment for sleep apnea, pushes pressurized air into your nose, keeping your airway open while you sleep. It prevents snoring and allows you to sleep deeply without frequent awakenings. Then, for the remainder of the night, they would observe how I did with the aid of CPAP.

Sleeping with Electrodes

I got to the Sleep Disorders Center at about 8 PM with my pajamas, pillow, and anything else that would put me at ease. I was told not to wear any makeup or use any conditioner in my hair so that the electrodes they would attach to my face and scalp would stay put.

After they showed me to my room, I watched a video about the CPAP machine; if I did have sleep apnea, I would be fitted with a mask attached to one of these machines during the night. After the video, I was outfitted with 14 different electrodes, which throughout the night would measure my brain waves; eye movements; muscle activity; chest, abdominal, and leg movements;

blood-oxygen saturation; snoring; and heart rate, as well as my nose and mouth breathing.

By 10 PM, I was pooped and ready for bed. Once the lights went out, a polysomnographic technologist would be watching me on a video monitor from another room, keeping track of the data my electrodes were sending out throughout the night.

Need I mention that it was *very* hard to sleep with all those electrodes secured to so many parts

Eight Steps to Better Sleep

You don't necessarily have to have a sleep disorder to be experiencing problems getting enough shuteye. Read the following list of habits that make for good "sleep hygiene," as the experts call it. Then look for a few you can change now to prevent future sleep problems. The closer you come to "perfect" sleep hygiene, the better you'll sleep every night.

1. Make sleep a priority.
2. Go to bed at the same time every night, and get up at the same time every morning.
3. Establish a soothing, relaxing routine to help you wind down before going to bed.
4. Avoid caffeine, alcohol, and smoking at least 3 hours before bed.
5. Keep the bedroom dark, cool, and quiet.
6. Exercise regularly.
7. Avoid the temptation to work, eat, or watch TV in bed.
8. Try replacing your afternoon coffee break with a 20-minute nap. Avoid playing catch-up with a 2-hour nap on the weekend.

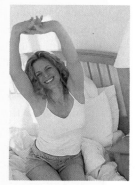

Good sleep means more good mornings.

If you adopt these healthy habits and still have trouble sleeping, make an appointment to discuss your concerns with your doctor. Sleep disturbances can also be a symptom of other problems, including hyperthyroidism, hypertension, restless legs syndrome, joint pain, an overactive bladder, certain drugs, and, as this chapter demonstrates, sleep apnea.

of my body, especially the thin, tickly wires that rested just inside my nostrils? I remember chastising myself, "If you don't get to sleep, they won't find out whether you have sleep apnea, and you'll either have to go through this again or continue feeling dead tired for the rest of your life." But somehow, magically, I did fall asleep. In fact, according to the sleep technologist, I had been snoozing even during that period of time when I'd been fretting about not falling asleep!

At 2 AM, a sleep technician came into my room to hook me up to the CPAP machine. I was so excited! Being fitted with the CPAP had to mean that I did have sleep apnea after all, and the CPAP would signal the death knell for my chronic sleep deprivation.

‖ The Results

Around 5:00 in the morning, the polysomnographic technologist came into my room and explained that they had enough information from the test to make a diagnosis. I left and returned to the center later to meet with Joe Schellenberg, MD, one of Dr. Strobel's colleagues at the Sleep Disorders Center.

Dr. Schellenberg explained that I did have obstructive sleep apnea, because I had stopped breathing during sleep. When I stopped, there had been a corresponding increase in brain wave activity at the end of the apneas (the arousals noted above). Without the CPAP machine, I had woken up about 16 times an hour without even realizing it! Even though 16 awakenings may seem like a lot—and believe me, it is enough to make a person feel miserable—I actually have a mild case of sleep apnea. People with severe cases can wake up hundreds of times a night!

‖ My Options

Since my sleep apnea is relatively mild, I had a greater number of treatment options than people with more severe cases. Dr. Schellenberg explained that CPAP is a cumbersome, lifelong treatment that must be used every time you sleep for maximum benefit. The upside? Insurance usually covers the cost.

Dr. Schellenberg told me about a special dental device that might aid in realigning my jaw, thus helping to keep my airway open as I slept. Unfortunately, the device costs approximately $500, was not guaranteed to work, and probably would not be covered by insurance.

My third option, said Dr. Schellenberg, was surgery. Still considered experimental by some experts, surgery isn't always successful. Equally important, the procedure can be quite painful. For me, the decision was an easy one to make: I chose CPAP.

‖ The Tinkering Begins

Immediately after meeting with Dr. Schellenberg, I was fitted with a nasal mask and was given a CPAP machine and a humidifier that would add moisture to the pressurized air. I assumed that from that point on, I would be enjoying the benefits of deep, restful sleep. But it didn't happen that way. In fact, the mask at first seemed to create more problems than it solved. For the first 2 to 3 weeks, my nights were replete with bothersome air leaks and the frustration that came with adjusting cumbersome tubing all night long.

Tired as I was, I decided to stick with the

therapy, come what may. So to deal with the tubing issue, my husband looped some string around the headboard of our bed through which the tube could pass, which gave me more turning leeway. Tubing problem solved.

But I still had other concerns. For one thing, I started snoring again. Because my mask covered only my nose, I was still breathing through my mouth. I wasn't getting the prescribed airflow to keep my airway open. To combat the problem, I tried a chin strap designed to keep my mouth closed. Unfortunately, the strap would slip off my chin throughout the night, making it virtually worthless.

So I returned to the medical supply company where I had gotten my CPAP, prepared to pay out of pocket for a full-face mask if that's what it would take to solve the problem once and for all. (My full-face mask covers both my nose and mouth, so no matter how I breathe, the air gets in.) In addition to giving me the full amount of air, the mask also fits me so well that I rarely have any annoying air leaks.

Because of my excellent care and treatment—all of which was covered by insurance—as well as my own stubborn persistence, I no longer snore. I'm happy to say that I sleep more deeply than I have in years! And my husband can finally sleep in our bed all night, every night.

CHAPTER 25

Does Your Body Have the Blues?

Gaining weight? Feeling tired? Can't relax? You may have women's most misdiagnosed mood problem

At any given time, tens of millions of women are troubled by a syndrome for which they have no name. A syndrome that leaves them feeling lethargic, tired, and craving snacks. A syndrome that leads to weight gain and a lack of motivation to exercise. Any of this sound familiar? Maybe you, too, have a case of this syndrome—the one that Marie-Annette Brown, PhD, calls the Body Blues.

To help women find a name and a treatment for this group of symptoms, Dr. Brown, a specialist in women's health care and adult mental health, along with bestselling *New York Times* health writer Jo Robinson, wrote a book called *When Your Body Gets the Blues* (Rodale Inc., 2002). Here is an excerpt from that book. Read on, and discover if your body's singing the

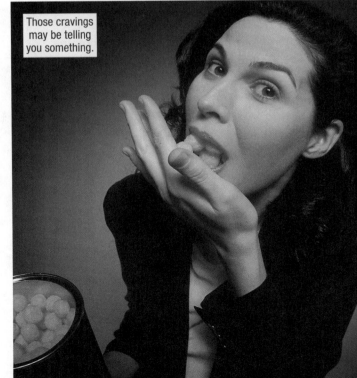

Those cravings may be telling you something.

blues—and how you can get it to whistle a healthier, happier tune.

A Case History of the Body Blues

Take one of my patients; I'll call her Joanne. She has four of the most common symptoms: fatigue, irritability, low sexual desire, and weight gain. To the casual observer, she appears to be a competent, confident woman who just happens to be slightly overweight.

Most nights she gets 7 to 8 hours of sleep, but by early afternoon, she is overwhelmed by the need to take a nap. Because her office is in her home, she can lie down whenever she needs to,

Do You Have the Body Blues?

A woman with the Body Blues will have three or more of the following symptoms:

▶ Eating too much and gaining weight

▶ Lack of energy

▶ Irritability or tension

▶ Difficulty concentrating

▶ Sleep problems

▶ Daytime drowsiness

▶ Decreased interest in sex

▶ Mild anxiety

▶ Mild depression

▶ Heightened sensitivity to rejection or criticism

but she resents taking the time. "I'm only 39," she told me. "I shouldn't have to take a nap!"

Joanne also feels stressed and irritable much of the time. "My employees and clients soak up most of my patience during the day," she explains. "My son gets what's left. And I'm much more critical of my husband than I want to be."

Even though Joanne listed fatigue as her reason for seeing me, I could tell she was even more concerned about her weight. At 5'6" and 172 lb, she's about 30 lb overweight. "I have no problem controlling what I eat for breakfast and lunch," she told me during our first appointment, "but everything falls apart in the late afternoon. I eat before, during, and after dinner. Now I'm back in my fat clothes."

Sleepy, Grumpy, and Snack Happy?

As a nurse practitioner at the University of Washington's Women's Health Care Center in Seattle, I've been trained to look at the whole person, not just her symptoms. I ordered blood tests for Joanne to rule out some of the common physical problems linked with fatigue, such as underactive thyroid, diabetes, and anemia. They all came back negative. I also interviewed her extensively and gave her several tests for underlying mood problems. As I had begun to suspect during her first appointment, Joanne is one of the millions of women with the most misdiagnosed, undertreated, and mistreated mood problem: the Body Blues.

One of the most common complaints is feeling tired and sluggish much of the time. To their dismay, women with the Body Blues often lack the energy to be the patient moms, supportive partners, or fun-loving friends they would like to

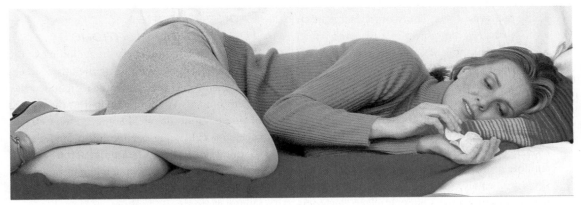

Do you have the four top Body Blues symptoms: fatigue, irritability, low sexual desire, and weight gain?

be. Although they know that exercise would help revive them, they rarely have the time or the motivation. Difficulty concentrating is another telltale sign, especially in women 35 and older. Trouble focusing on tasks, absorbing complex information, and remembering names can be a source of embarrassment.

But the most common and vexing symptoms of all are overeating and weight gain. Like Joanne, most women with the Body Blues have little trouble controlling their appetite in the morning. But sometime in the afternoon, they begin to snack. A craving for sweets and starches is one of the defining characteristics of this syndrome.

You might expect women with this disorder to have serious mood problems. But they don't. Unlike women with clinical depression, women with the Body Blues don't feel sad or tearful most of the time. When something good happens to them, they feel genuinely happy. Nonetheless, they can be very distressed by their fatigue, eating problems, irritability, confused thinking, or sleep

difficulties. These symptoms interfere with relationships, frustrate ambitions, and rob women of the full enjoyment of life. It's as though their bodies were depressed, but not their minds.

Why Women Are at Risk

Many of my patients think that their symptoms are caused by a lack of willpower, laziness, or sheer gluttony. This is rarely the case. In the past 10 years, scientists have learned that every symptom of the Body Blues can be traced back to some aspect of a woman's physiology. Here's how women's hormonal swings contribute.

Estrogen: The Energetic Hormone

Low or falling estrogen levels are one of the main triggers of the Body Blues. Estrogen rises from the lowest to the highest level during the first 2 weeks of the menstrual cycle. This monthly surge influences virtually every aspect of a woman's being, including her supply of serotonin, the brain's primary feel-good chemical.

When estrogen levels are high, women have more serotonin activity in the brain. Greater serotonin activity is linked to better mood, reduced appetite, more physical energy, and more resilience to stress. This makes serotonin a potent antidote to the Body Blues.

Estrogen also increases the amount of blood that flows to a woman's brain. It relaxes key arteries, allowing more blood to pass through. When cerebral bloodflow is high, people have better memories and are less likely to be depressed.

When estrogen levels are low or falling, women have less serotonin activity. Women have low levels of estrogen in the days before menstruation, after giving birth, while breastfeeding, during perimenopause, and during the years following menopause. These are the very times when they are most likely to have the Body Blues.

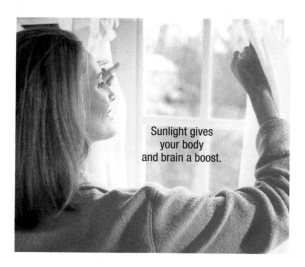

Sunlight gives
your body
and brain a boost.

Progesterone: The Calming Hormone

Progesterone also influences the symptoms of the Body Blues. High levels during the final 2 weeks of the menstrual cycle may cause a slight decrease in serotonin activity in the brain. But these levels of progesterone do yield some positive effects, including enhancing sleep, calming anxiety, and soothing irritability. When progesterone falls off at the end of the cycle, women lose its tranquilizing, sleep-enhancing properties and are thus more vulnerable to the Body Blues.

Testosterone: The Pleasure Hormone

Testosterone is the hormone that fuels sexual desire and enhances pleasure—in women as well as men. As is true for estrogen and progesterone, testosterone levels also vary across the menstrual cycle. Testosterone is low during the first part of the cycle, peaks at ovulation, and then declines during the final 2 weeks of the cycle. When a woman has relatively high levels, she is more likely to think about sex, respond to a partner's advances, and initiate sex. There is growing evidence that some symptoms of depression and the Body Blues, especially fatigue, anxiety, and low sexual desire, may be due to a woman's variable supply of testosterone.

Are You Getting Enough Light?

It's not just fluctuating hormones that bring on the Body Blues; light deprivation can contribute as well. The more time you spend in low light conditions, the more likely you will feel tired, eat too much, gain weight, and feel drowsy during the day, all of which are key symptoms of the Body Blues.

Most people underestimate the difference in light levels between indoors and out. Surprisingly, there is as much as 1,000 times more light available to us once we step outside. Surveys show that most of us spend a whopping 23 hours a day indoors. As soon as we leave our home in the morning, we duck into a car, bus, or train. When we arrive at work, we scurry inside. After work, we run a few errands and then hurry back home. Then we spend most of our evenings cocooning indoors: reading, watching TV, catching up on paperwork, or being "mouse potatoes," slang for those of us who've become addicted to our computers. As a result, we get just a fraction of the light our bodies require. Surveys show that women get even less light than men.

Your 20-Minute Prescription

You can beat the Body Blues in just 20 minutes a day by following a clinically proven, scientifically sound program developed by me and my colleagues at the University of Washington. It's called the LEVITY program, a drug-free solution based on three commonsense activities:

1. Creating a more natural lighting environment
2. Going for a brisk 20-minute outdoor walk, five or more times a week
3. Taking six common and inexpensive vitamins and minerals

The success of our program was graphically demonstrated by a study at the university that was

---

DO JUST ONE THING!

Light Up Your Life

Here are a number of ways to light up your environment. Identify those that seem most practical and helpful for you, and plan to act upon them within a week.

- ▶ **Go for outdoor walks five or more times a week.**
- ▶ **Look straight ahead rather than down at the ground when you walk. A level gaze can more than double the amount of light that enters your eyes.**
- ▶ **Use a transparent umbrella when it rains or snows.**
- ▶ **Wear lightly tinted sunglasses to block ultraviolet light but let in all the mood-boosting visible light.**
- ▶ **Open the blinds or curtains while you're home.**
- ▶ **Rearrange your furniture to face the windows.**
- ▶ **Paint walls a brighter color.**
- ▶ **Add windows, skylights, glass doors, or a sunroom.**
- ▶ **Install the brightest lightbulbs your lamps will safely allow.**
- ▶ **Choose window seats in cars, buses, planes, trains, and other transportation devices, whenever possible.**
- ▶ **Plan a winter vacation in a sunny location.**

published in the journal *Women & Health* in 2001. In just 8 weeks, the women who took part in the program felt more energetic, reduced their appetites, began thinking more clearly, and had a more positive sense of well-being. On one of the tests, their depression scores were cut in half!

Why does the program work? Getting more bright light, engaging in moderate intensity exercise, and taking the right vitamins and minerals reverses many of the physical changes brought about by low or fluctuating hormones and living a light-deprived existence. These three activities boost serotonin activity in your brain, increase your cerebral bloodflow, and reduce your stress hormones.

Step 1: Recharge Your Solar Batteries

There are three ways that bright light can help relieve the Body Blues. First, when sunlight falls on your bare skin, your body produces more vitamin D, a vitamin with proven mood-elevating properties. Second, when light enters your eyes, it triggers the production of a variety of feel-good chemicals. Third, bright light increases bloodflow to your brain, which relieves depression and helps you with concentration and memory. Studies have confirmed that brightening your environment boosts physical energy, helps you sleep better at night, and stimulates bloodflow to the brain to boost mood and relieve confused thinking.

There's one additional benefit of getting more bright light that has gotten very little media attention: Bright light alone can help you lose weight in the following four ways:

▶ Lifts your spirits, which reduces your need to self-medicate with food
▶ Increases your activity level, which helps you burn more calories
▶ Suppresses your appetite, which lowers your caloric intake
▶ Helps boost your metabolism

Until modern times, women got all the benefits of bright light simply by going about their normal routines. But today, we have to consciously seek out the sun. All the billions of dollars that people spend on diet programs might be better spent on skylights, sunrooms, outdoor recreation, and all-weather walking gear.

Don't Exceed These Daily Upper Limits

Thiamin	100 mg
Riboflavin	200 mg
Vitamin B$_6$	100 mg
Folic acid	1,000 mcg
Vitamin D	2,000 IU
Selenium	400 mcg

In proper doses, these nutrients are a healthy "cocktail."

Step 2: Walk Away from the Body Blues

New research reveals that you don't have to break a sweat to get mood-enhancing benefits from exercise. Nor do you have to join an expensive gym, buy special equipment, put on a skimpy leotard, or even change your clothes. All you need to do is put on a pair of comfortable shoes, open the door, and start walking.

Imagine that you've just stepped out the door and started to walk. You are swinging your arms and aiming for a pace that is midway between a stroll and a jog. As your heart rate increases, more blood flows to your brain. The increased bloodflow enhances your ability to think and concentrate.

At the same time, the brisk walk revs up your body, triggering the release of the same activating substances brought on by stress. But the amounts generated by walking make you feel energized and alert, not tense and irritable. In technical terms, walking produces an "energetic arousal" rather than a "tense arousal."

Though many women turn to food to relieve their anxiety, low mood, and fatigue, walking is a much better way to ease tension, reduce anxiety, and help buffer yourself against stress. (You'll find three great walking programs to choose from in Chapter 8.)

A brisk 20-minute walk outdoors, 5 days a week, offers these benefits:

▶ Increases your energy level
▶ Increases the serotonin activity in your brain
▶ Connects you with nature
▶ Burns fat
▶ Decreases your appetite
▶ Reduces your risk of heart disease, stroke, diabetes, osteoporosis, and high blood pressure

1-MINUTE *HEALTH BOOSTER*

Overcome Your Exercise Inertia

Do you have doubts that you'll be able to motivate yourself to go for frequent walks? The good news is that the more sedentary you are, the more you'll benefit physically and mentally from exercise. But first you need to overcome your inertia and find ways to look forward to your 20-minute exercise session. To do that, circle the letters of the activities below that will make your exercise session more appealing to you. Then write down how you plan to put them into action.

A. Exercise by myself so I can be free of the demands of other people and think my own thoughts.

B. Exercise with a group of friends.

C. Listen to my favorite music.

D. Listen to educational or inspirational tapes.

E. Walk in a beautiful setting.

F. Use a pedometer or heart rate monitor.

G. Have a destination such as a friend's house or local store.

H. Walk a dog.

I. Discover new parts of the city.

J. Come home, and treat myself to a favorite ritual, such as drinking a hot cup of tea and reading the paper, or taking a soak in the tub.

Step 3: Take Your Antidepressant Cocktail

Brightening your indoor environment and going for regular brisk walks outside can jump-start the production of a number of mood-enhancing, stress-relieving, and appetite-suppressing chemicals. But your body cannot manufacture those chemicals unless it has the raw ingredients necessary to make them.

The third and final component of the LEVITY program supplies these essential ingredients. When you add this antidepressant "cocktail" to a program of bright light and moderate-intensity exercise, you have our clinically proven remedy for the Body Blues.

While nutrient/mood research is still in its infancy, enough reliable information exists about the safety and effectiveness of these six nutrients that I've made them an integral part of our program.

Thiamin (vitamin B₁), 50 mg: relieves fatigue and improves memory

Riboflavin (vitamin B₂), 50 mg: essential for the regular production of the mood boosting chemicals serotonin, dopamine, and norepinephrine

Vitamin B₆ (pyridoxine), 50 mg: stimulates serotonin production

Folic acid, 400 micrograms (mcg): helps relieve depression

Vitamin D (cholecalciferol), 400 IU: stimulates production of serotonin

Selenium, 200 mcg: enhances the dopamine activity in the brain, increasing sense of arousal and pleasure

Taking your daily supplements will be the easiest part of the LEVITY program. It requires just a few seconds of your time. The only work involved is deciding what you need to buy and then developing a simple strategy to make sure you take the tablets regularly. If you are taking nutritional supplements already, check how much thiamin, riboflavin, B₆, folic acid, vitamin D, and selenium you're getting. And make sure that adding these above amounts to your current regimen will not put you above the safe limits. (See "Don't Exceed These Daily Upper Limits" on p. 182.)

Your Everyday Health Planner
Use this quick reference to help you adopt healthier habits—now!

It can be tough to make sure you're doing everything you can to preserve your health. But every little bit adds up! Here are 20 habits that will help you feel better every day of your life, along with references to chapters that can help you implement them. Make it your goal to add one new healthy habit each week. The more you check off, the better you'll feel!

❑ **1.** I don't "medicate" emotions with food. (Chapter 1)

❑ **2.** I eat healthy, satisfying meals and snacks. (Chapter 2)

❑ **3.** I take appropriate vitamin and mineral supplements. (Chapter 5)

❑ **4.** I eat nine servings of fruits and vegetables each day. (Chapter 6)

❑ **5.** I strength-train regularly. (Chapter 7)

❑ **6.** I go for a walk nearly every day. (Chapter 8)

❑ **7.** I keep belly fat to a minimum. (Chapter 9)

❑ **8.** I take time to stretch and relax. (Chapter 10)

❑ **9.** I am aware of my genetic risk factors for major health conditions. (Chapter 11)

❑ **10.** I know my cholesterol level and do all I can to keep it in check. (Chapter 12)

❑ **11.** I do all I can to keep my cancer risk to a minimum. (Chapter 13)

❑ **12.** I know my blood sugar level and do all I can to prevent diabetes. (Chapter 14)

❑ **13.** I do all I can to protect my bones from osteoporosis. (Chapter 16)

❑ **14.** I get an annual gynecological exam, examine my breasts monthly, and get mammograms when my doctor recommends it. (Chapters 17 and 18)

❑ **15.** I notify my doctor whenever I notice new symptoms of any sort, including but not limited to joint pain, menstrual changes, and heart palpitations. (Chapter 19)

❑ **16.** I consult with my doctor before taking supplements, herbs, or over-the-counter medicines and before I make any changes involving a prescription medication. (Chapter 20)

❑ **17.** I discuss sexual concerns (and enjoyment!) with my partner openly and honestly. (Chapter 21)

❑ **18.** I practice good "sleep hygiene." (Chapter 24)

❑ **19.** I set aside some time every day just for me. (Chapter 26)

❑ **20.** I try to be optimistic about myself, my life, and my future. (Chapter 28)

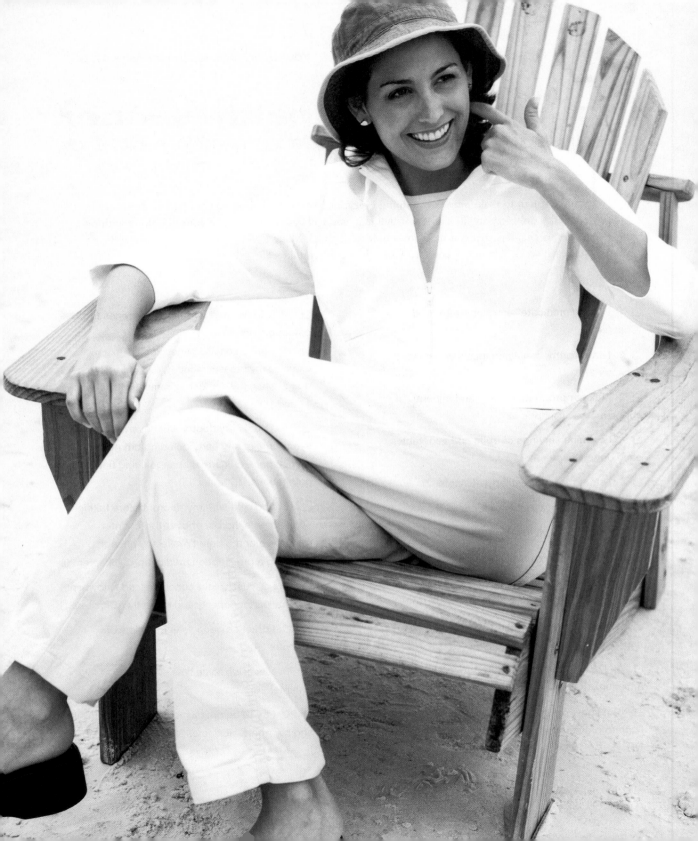

Soothe Your Soul

Create 15 Days of Free Time

Can't find an hour to yourself? Here's how to reclaim 365 of them this year!

As every woman knows, there's already not enough time in a day to pick up the kids after soccer, take your mother to the doctor, put in a full day's work, drop the dog at the vet, listen to your husband rehash his day, make dinner, help the kids with homework, and still take a walk, nap, or just plain breathe. Does it have to be like this just because you're a woman? Fortunately, the answer is a resounding "no."

"Women usually define success by how they connect with people," explains Lenora Yuen, PhD, a psychologist in Palo Alto, CA. So to be the "perfect" woman, you need to be a good friend, a good mother, a good everything. Unfortunately, that means that if you decide to go to yoga class instead of listening to a friend moan about her husband, you'll feel like

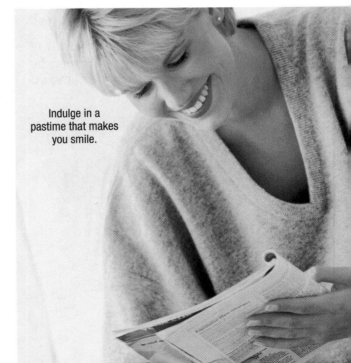

Indulge in a pastime that makes you smile.

you're not being a good friend, a good woman, or even a decent human being.

If you're never too busy to help someone else with their life—even if that means *you* don't get to have a life, you suffer from what Los Angeles psychologist Harriet Braiker, PhD, calls "the disease to please. People pleasers just can't say no. As a result, their time is filled with compulsively meeting the needs of others. They expect to make time for themselves *after* they've taken care of everybody else, but they never get to themselves."

Sound familiar? Here's how to learn to turn the spotlight on *you* a little more.

Ditch the Time Wasters

Stress, perfectionism, people pleasing, and the demands of life in the 21st century are pretty big obstacles to overcome on your own. Yet if you deal with them effectively, you can reclaim an hour a day for yourself.

Give the following suggestions a try. By this time next year, you'll have gotten back a whopping 15 days in which to do whatever you please.

Analyze your time wasters. Everybody has at least one. The key is to figure out what yours is, then refuse to make it a recurring appointment in your date book. For example, if you're always rummaging around trying to find objects, then you need to get rid of the clutter and get organized—even if that means hiring someone to help you.

Stop saying yes. "Learning to say no is probably the one key skill to overcoming people pleasing," says Dr. Braiker. If you have trouble

Identify What's Draining You

What's keeping you from finding 1 measly hour each day for yourself? See if any of these scenarios sound familiar.

▶ You have too much going on to think straight. You're so stressed out that you can't focus on what you're doing. So you end up wasting time looking for lost car keys, searching for misplaced papers, and trying to remember what you went into the living room to retrieve.

▶ You're always running from home to work to the dry cleaner to school to work to home, and you simply haven't taken the time to figure out what you'd do if you had any free time.

▶ You don't have time for you because it's all used up by everyone else. You're afraid that if you take time for yourself, you won't be able to do all the things you expect of yourself. You're afraid you won't be perfect.

Do any (or all) of these sound familiar? If so, you don't have to be locked into these draining behaviors. Try the tips in this chapter to break the cycle starting *today*.

doing it, try to buy a little time before responding. Answer every request with "Let me think about that and check my schedule."

Don't take detours. Run through today's schedule, and list all the things that distracted you from doing what you really intended to do, says Chicago therapist Maryann Troiani, PhD, author of *Spontaneous Optimism: Proven Strategies for Health, Prosperity and Happiness* (Castlegate, 1998). Maybe there was a television program you never meant to watch or a link to a Web site you never intended to visit—especially not at 1:00 AM. Resolve not to let yourself get sucked in again.

Bring technology under control. "So many professional people start checking their voice mail on Sunday night," says Dr. Troiani. Or they read their e-mail to find out what to expect

the next day. That not only robs you of downtime, she points out, but it cuts into the quality of time you spend with others. Use technology to make your life easier—not to expand the workday.

Be ruthless. "Make a list of everything you do for a month," says Dr. Braiker, who is also the author of *The Disease to Please* (McGraw-Hill, 2001). Then, assign 10% of everything on the list to someone else to do. Ask yourself "Is there anything on this list that's essential for me to do myself?" If there is, says Dr. Braiker, keep it. Is there anything on the list that gives you pleasure or cre-

DO JUST ONE THING!

Cure Clutter-itis!

You haven't seen your kitchen table or desktop in months because of all the clutter that has accumulated: coupons, receipts, directions —all missing in action. Finding what you need, when you need it, is impossible!

The best way to get rid of clutter forever is to come up with a way to get organized that matches your personality, needs, and goals. Try these tips from Julie Morgenstern, author of *Organizing from the Inside Out* (Henry Holt and Company, 1998).

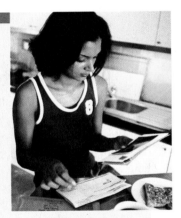

Set daily goals: Decide exactly how and when you'll treat yourself.

1. Follow the kindergarten model of organizing, which can be applied to your entire home, one room, or just a drawer. Divide the space into activity zones that reflect how you use that space. Group like items together within a zone, and choose storage units that work best in the space.

2. Choose a regular time every day, and spend 15 to 30 minutes going through mail, taking care of paperwork, or just putting things away. If you wait until you have a "free minute," it won't get done and will allow clutter to build up.

3. Choose storage containers that you love and are fun to use and look at. You'll be more motivated to use them.

For more tips, check out *The New Messies Manual* by Sandra Felton (Fleming H. Revell, 2000) and *Stephanie Winston's Best Organizing Tips* (Simon & Schuster/Fireside, 1996).

ates meaning in your life? Keep that too. Anything that stresses you out should be a top choice for delegating. Just don't be fussy about how others do the tasks that you relinquish, cautions Dr. Braiker. "You can't get time back unless you realize that it's more important for somebody else to do the job than it is for the job to be done exactly your way."

Get rid of emotional vampires. "We want cheerleaders in our life," says Dr. Troiani. "We don't want those drainers and complainers who take up all our time and suck us dry. Complainers usually have one issue that they repeat 10 times. So when a complainer starts in, listen once, and say, 'I hear you. Now what are you going to do about it?'" Help them brainstorm if you'd like. But if they don't start coming up with solutions, it's time for you to make an exit.

‖ Rebuild Your Day

Once you've reclaimed an hour a day for yourself, you're ready to do some serious thinking about how you're going to make it happen on a regular basis. Here's what our experts suggest.

Find your vision. Many times people can't find an extra hour to do something because the something really isn't what they want to do, says Dr. Troiani. For example, when the husband of one of Dr. Troiani's clients wanted his wife to lose weight, the woman just couldn't find the time to exercise. After talking to her, Dr. Troiani realized why: She didn't really want to lose weight, so the exercise just never happened.

That's why you have to sit down, reflect, and feel in your heart what it is you want to find time for, says Dr. Troiani. "You need to ask yourself 'Is this what I really want to do?' and 'How will I feel in 5 years if I don't do it?'"

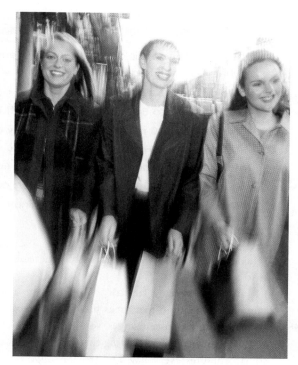

Taking time for yourself isn't selfish—it makes you more fun to be with!

Set goals. Once you decide what you want to do, determine exactly what day you will do it and at what time. For instance, if you want to go for outdoor walks more often, plan to do it every Saturday morning. Once you're into the routine, you may want to add one weekday morning too. A few months later, maybe you'll find yourself walking every morning.

Start with 15 minutes. It's hard for anyone to dig an hour or two of free time out of a busy life. So write 15 minutes into your

Your "Time-for-Myself" Daily Goals

To make sure you stick to your plan to spend more time on *you,* here's a quick reminder of what you need to do each day:

▶ Avoid time wasters. (See p. 189.)

▶ Schedule 15 to 60 minutes to yourself; be specific about what you'll do when.

▶ Spend 15 to 30 minutes clearing away clutter. (See p. 190.)

▶ Say "no" to unimportant requests; say "I'll get back to you" to buy time before making a decision on ones you're not sure about.

▶ Stop working when your shift is over; don't take work home.

▶ Write in your worry journal for 15 minutes (see below), then put your worries aside.

schedule, says Dr. Yuen. Then gradually increase it to an hour.

Take a worry break. Worry can be a constant companion that sucks up energy when you're trying to make changes, so give it a place to go by journaling everything that worries you for 15 minutes every day, Dr. Troiani suggests. Then put away the journal—and the worries.

Set deadlines. If you procrastinate about taking time for yourself, say "Okay, by Monday, I

will have taken an hour to . . . ." Deadlines defeat procrastination every time, says Dr. Troiani.

Retrain family and friends. Everyone you've showered with your time is now thoroughly spoiled. Be prepared for them to be disappointed when you start to reserve a little time for yourself, says Dr. Yuen. "It doesn't make you a bad or selfish person to take a couple of hours," she adds. In the long run, it'll probably make you a lot more fun to be with.

CHAPTER 27

Your Secret Weapon against Stress

Scientists say that bonding with our girlfriends can release calming hormones

Friendships between women are special. They shape who we are and who we are yet to be. They soothe our tumultuous inner world, fill the emotional gaps in our marriage, and help us remember who we really are. And now research suggests that they may be able to do even more. Scientists now suspect that hanging out with our friends can actually counteract the kind of nerve-jangling stress that many of us experience on a daily basis.

That's right: Women researchers have discovered that women respond differently to stress than men do—namely by seeking each other's company. Read on for the science that illuminated the importance of female friendships, along with tips for helping you give these relationships the attention they deserve.

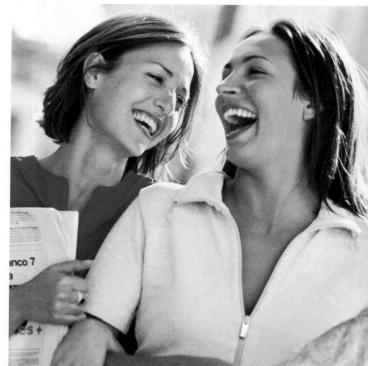

Friends are a unique source of strength.

How Friendship Zaps Stress

A landmark UCLA study suggests that women respond to stress with a cascade of brain chemicals that cause them to make and maintain friendships with other women. It's a stunning finding that has turned 5 decades of stress research—most of it on men—upside down.

"Until this study was published, scientists generally believed that when people experience stress, they trigger a hormonal cascade that revs the

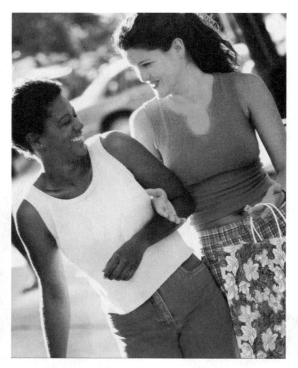

Friendships may lengthen your lifespan by buffering you from the negative effects of stress.

body to either stand and fight or flee as fast as possible," explains Laura Cousino Klein, PhD, now an assistant professor of biobehavioral health at Pennsylvania State University in State College and one of the study's authors. It's an ancient survival mechanism left over from the time we were chased across the planet by saber-toothed tigers. And it's a theory based largely on research on men. Now researchers suspect that women have a larger behavioral repertoire than just "fight or flight."

In fact, says Dr. Klein, it seems that when the hormone oxytocin is released as part of the stress response in a woman, it buffers the fight or flight response and encourages her to tend children and gather with other women instead. When she actually engages in this tending or befriending, studies suggest that more oxytocin is released, which further counters stress and produces a calming effect.

This calming response does not occur in men, says Dr. Klein, because testosterone—which men produce in high levels when they're under stress—seems to reduce the effects of oxytocin. Estrogen, she adds, seems to enhance it.

Women Scientists Make the Connection

The discovery that women respond to stress differently than men was made in a classic "aha!" moment shared by two women scientists who were talking one day in a lab at UCLA.

"There was this joke that when the women who worked in the lab were stressed, they came in, cleaned the lab, had coffee, and bonded," says Dr. Klein. "When the men were stressed, they holed up somewhere on their own."

1-MINUTE *STRESS BUSTER*

Eat to Beat Anxiety

A stressful day could send anyone on the hunt for chocolate, but if you regularly reach for ice cream, cookies, or cake when you're upset or tense, it may have nothing to do with a lack of willpower. For you, carbohydrates may stimulate an especially powerful release of pleasure-producing hormones in your body. Like a nicotine addiction, such a compulsion is tough to break—but not impossible. Surprisingly, food can help you do it. Sweet-but-nutritious complex carbohydrates such as the foods listed below have the same calming effect. However, they're less harmful to your waistline, because they have fewer calories than the candy bars or other calorie-rich foods you might normally seek, explains Leigh Gibson, PhD, a senior research fellow at University College London who has studied this phenomenon.

You'll also be less likely to overeat throughout the rest of the day if you treat your choice like a meal instead of a mindless snack. Find a place away from your office or away from whoever is upsetting you. Then sit down, and slowly enjoy your food.

Foods for Stress-Induced Cravings

- ▶ Fresh fruit or canned light fruit
- ▶ Lightly sweetened whole grain cereals such as Multi-Grain Cheerios
- ▶ Multi grain waffle with light syrup
- ▶ Oatmeal
- ▶ Sweet potato, or baked potato with light sour cream and chives
- ▶ Tomato soup
- ▶ Whole wheat toast with jam

"I commented one day to fellow researcher Shelley Taylor that nearly 90% of the stress research is on males. I showed her the data from my lab, and the two of us knew instantly that we were onto something." The women cleared their schedules and started meeting with one scientist after another from various research specialties.

Very quickly, Drs. Klein and Taylor discovered that by not including women in stress research, scientists had made a huge mistake: The fact that women respond to stress differently than men has significant implications for our health.

How Friends Can Save Your Life

It may take some time for new studies to reveal all the ways that oxytocin encourages us to care for children and hang out with other women, but the "tend and befriend" notion developed by Drs. Klein and Taylor may explain why women consistently outlive men. Study after study has found that social ties reduce our risk of disease by lowering blood pressure, heart rate, and cholesterol. There's no doubt, says Dr. Klein, that friends are helping us live longer.

In one study, for example, researchers found that people who had no friends increased their risk of death over a 6-month period. In another study, those who had the most friends over a 9-year period cut their risk of death by more than 60%.

Friends are also helping us live *better*. The

DO JUST ONE THING!

Bring Your Friends to Work

Studies have shown that people in high-stress jobs often don't realize they're stressed. You could be one of them. One quick way to ease workday tension is to make your desk or office feel more like home. Display framed snapshots of your friends goofing around, and hang photos of your family near your computer monitor. Bring in a few souvenirs from your last vacation with the gang, and decorate your desk. These personal touches can help relax you even on your busiest day.

---

famed Nurses' Health Study from Harvard Medical School found that the more friends women had, the less likely they were to develop physical impairments as they aged, and the more likely they were to be leading a joyful life. In fact, the results were so significant, the researchers concluded, that *not* having a close friend or confidante was as detrimental to your health as smoking or carrying extra weight!

And that's not all: When the researchers looked at how well the women functioned after the death of their spouse, they found that even in the face of this biggest stressor of all, those women who had a close friend and confidante were more likely to survive the experience without any new physical impairment or permanent loss of vitality.

Putting Friends First

If friends counter the stress that's so prevalent these days, if they keep us healthy and even add years to our lives, why is it so hard to find time to be with them? That's a question that also troubles researcher Ruthellen Josselson, PhD, coauthor of *Best Friends: The Pleasures and Perils of Girls' and Women's Friendships* (Three Rivers Press, 1998). "Every time we get overly busy with work and family, the first thing we do is let go of friendships with other women," explains Dr. Josselson. "We push them right to the back burner. That's really a mistake, because women are such a source of strength to each other. We nurture one another. And we need to have unpressured space in which we can do the special kind of talk that women do when they're with other women. It's a very healing experience."

One way to make sure your friendships don't get the short shrift: Schedule time with them. Be formal about it. Put it on your calendar. If it helps

What's Saving You?

According to *Prevention* advisor Edward M. Hallowell, MD, a psychiatrist, an instructor at Harvard, and author of eight books, the main thing that gets us through life's toughest times is something he calls "human moments." "Human moments are moments of connection blossoming forth to give you a feeling of strength, safety, power, and hope," says Dr. Hallowell.

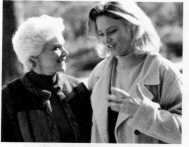

Maintaining strong bonds is as important for women as maintaining a healthy weight.

Have you ever wondered who—or what—saved you? The question may take you aback, especially if you didn't have to overcome any great obstacles in your past. But chances are *someone* helped bring you to where you are. Maybe it was a schoolteacher. Maybe it was your mother. Maybe it was a business partner or a doctor who made the right diagnosis. We like to think we save ourselves. We like to think that we can do it all, that we are independent. But no one is.

"What saves us all, but faith, hope, and love?" Dr. Hallowell asks. "Even if our faith is not in a God, it is faith that someone will be there when we get home, or faith that a loved one will be true to us. What saved me were other people—their love—and the faith and hope that kindled in me. Can you think of what is saving you?"

you to stick to your "dates," join something together that costs money, such as a yoga or pottery class. Or ask a friend to be your walking buddy. This way you'll get a dose of stress-busting friend time along with your calorie-burning workout.

And always be on the lookout for new opportunities to make connections. Life changes, job changes, and other unplanned events can cause old friends to fade out of our lives, so be sure to let new ones find their way in.

CHAPTER 28

Turn On Your Internal Optimist

Keep your mood sunny—and boost your health in the process

Has anyone ever told you to lighten up? Or is that something you hear on a fairly regular basis? Either way, ditching a pessimistic viewpoint is good for you.

New research shows that being happy-go-lucky can actually help preserve your health, says Carl J. Charnetski, PhD, a full professor and former chairman of the psychology department at Wilkes University in Wilkes-Barre, PA, and Francis X. Brennan, PhD, associate director of the Neurobehavioral Research Laboratory at the Department of Veterans Affairs Medical Center in East Orange, NJ. To help you turn *your* frown upside down, Drs. Charnetski and Brennan wrote the optimism-encouraging book *Feeling Good Is Good for You: How Pleasure Can Boost Your Immunity* (Rodale Inc., 2001), excerpted here.

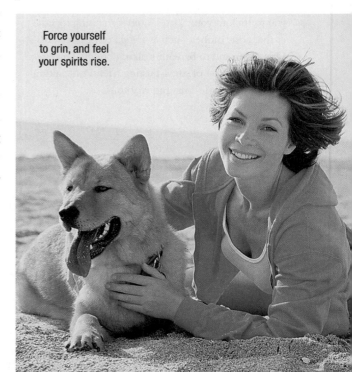

Force yourself to grin, and feel your spirits rise.

How Do *You* Look at Life?

The unique way that you view life—be it with an optimistic or pessimistic spin—is called your "explanatory style." Your explanatory style is composed of three very specific questions that you must ask yourself about whatever happens to you:

▶ Is the incident your fault?

▶ Is it temporary or long lasting?

▶ Does the cause affect one or many aspects of your life?

People can blend explanatory styles and fall anywhere between the two extremes of optimist and pessimist. But when something bad happens, pessimists tend to blame themselves. They believe that the cause of the bad event will be around for quite some time and that it will affect many parts of their life. Optimists, on the other hand, are essentially the opposite: They don't blame themselves, they expect the consequences to be minor and of short duration, and they don't let it affect other parts of their life.

How Your Style Affects Your Health

Unfortunately, how you wander through the world—either as an optimist or a pessimist—affects your health. Significantly.

Pessimists end up being sick more days in any given month than their more optimistic counterparts, according to a recent study done at the University of Michigan in Ann Arbor. Pessimists also go to the doctor more frequently.

Why? Well, that's what we wanted to know

1-MINUTE STRESS BUSTER

Give Yourself the Optimist Test

Are you an optimist or pessimist? Here's a quick way to find out.

Recall the most recent negative event you experienced in your life, and ask yourself why it happened.

Next, consider the most recent positive occurrence, and ask the same question.

If you attribute the negative event to your own stupidity or to the dark cloud that always seems to hover overhead, you are leaning toward the pessimistic side of life. If you chalk up the positive event to a stroke of dumb luck that probably won't happen again, you are also displaying a pessimistic nature.

too. The fact that pessimistic students in the study got colds and the flu more frequently than optimistic students suggested to us that IgA, a disease-fighting antibody that circulates in saliva and other body fluids, was somehow involved. (Low IgA levels correlate with getting sick.) So we decided to test the proposition.

In 1999, we gave the Attributional Style Questionnaire (ASQ)—devised to ferret out explanatory styles—to 116 students at Wilkes University in Wilkes-Barre, PA. While the students answered questions, we took saliva samples from them to check for the presence of IgA. No relationship existed between the overall scores and IgA or between optimism and IgA. However, the more pessimistic the students were or the more hopeless they felt, the lower their IgA.

Feeling Good Is Good for You

Why would a dark outlook on life have an influence on health? Perhaps pessimism and hopelessness cause IgA levels to drop. Maybe pessimists feel more stress and its attendant immune effects as they wait for disaster to strike. Maybe they just can't sit back, relax, and enjoy life. Maybe it's a combination. Or maybe it's something that science has yet to identify.

What is clear is that the worse you feel about yourself and the worse your outlook on life, the worse your health may be. You don't have to be a certified cynic or a dictionary definition of a depressed person. Day-to-day, hour-to-hour fluctuations in mood also exert an influence on your immune strength and on the odds that you'll get sick.

For instance, you might be a generally carefree, cheery, and well-adjusted person, but if you happen to be angry, upset, or otherwise negative just minutes before you run your hand along a stairway railing that harbors a flu virus, you're more likely to get a cold than if you were happy-go-lucky and free of hostility when you came into contact with the bug. That's because when you're angry, upset, or moody, even for a little while, your IgA drops markedly and your T lymphocytes slow to a crawl. (T lymphocytes are important immune system cells that include helper and killer T cells.)

Fine-Tune Your Attitude

But what if you're feeling bad? Are you doomed to an unhappy, unhealthy life? Of course not! No one feels good all of the time. But here are some ways to improve your mood when you're down and, in the process, boost your immunity.

Just do it. Even if you don't feel like getting off the couch, taking a shower, and going to the theater to see that movie you thought might be good, do it anyway.

Most of us think that attitude must change before behavior changes. That's true, but the inverse works also. If you force yourself to behave in a way that's out of sync with how you actually feel, your brain will change your attitude to come into accordance with your behavior.

Dump the doubters. Minimize the time you spend with complainers, doubters, and other pessimists. Try to think of negativity as the emotional equivalent of a room filled with cigarette smoke. Pessimism is a psychologically contagious disease.

Vent. This is crucial. Vent your repressed, emotionally charged feelings. At least once a week, visit with or call a different friend or family member, and talk about something that's been bothering you. Cycle through your list of confidantes, then start all over again.

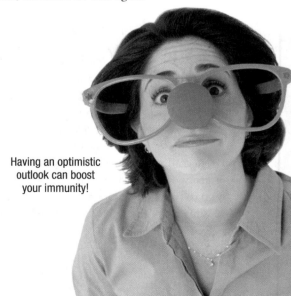

Having an optimistic outlook can boost your immunity!

DO JUST ONE THING !

Avoid On-the-Job Pessimism

When a project blows up at work, what do you do?

- (a) acknowledge that the project's success wasn't entirely dependent on your performance
- (b) always take complete responsibility for the snafu
- (c) conclude that you're not qualified for your job, and dismiss all previous successes as flukes

Answers: If you chose (a), your work attitude is healthy. If you chose (b), you need to start with realistic expectations. Before beginning a project, ask yourself if you have enough control to single-handedly guarantee its success. (That's almost never the case for anyone.) You'll be less likely to blame yourself if something goes awry. If you chose (c), you should credit yourself with past successes. Remind yourself regularly of past achievements—recall your yearly evaluations with your boss, or reread written evaluations—and give yourself credit where it's due.

Grin—it helps you bear it. Whether or not you have reason to do so, smile frequently. The nerves connected to your face's smile muscles project right into parts of the brain that help determine mood. Send a signal to your brain that you're happy, and "voilà!" you are happy—and so is your immune system.

Give yourself a round of applause. If something good happens, give yourself the credit you deserve. Make a big deal out of it. But when something unfortunate occurs, don't dwell on it. Don't bad-mouth yourself.

Get on a winning streak. Nothing succeeds like success, so set yourself up for a string of victories. Put yourself into situations that can have only positive outcomes. As you experience success, you'll begin to perceive yourself as successful, and your perception of yourself then dictates your behavior.

Plan to prolong pleasure. If you do something spontaneously on Saturday night, you

and your immune system will enjoy it—but only on Saturday night. But if you plan the activity on Thursday, you'll look forward to the enjoyment all day Thursday, all day Friday, and all day Saturday. Anticipating a positive event brightens your mood and attitude.

Take control. It's amazing how much of your life you can control if you think about it. Even if a situation is bad, exert some control. Don't wait all day for a confrontational phone call. Make the call at 9 AM instead of getting to it at 1 PM and suffering 4 hours of anticipatory anxiety. Your immune system hates this.

Focus on the positive. Don't dwell on the negative things that you have no control over. At any point, 90% of your life may be a mess and uncontrollable. Focus 90% of your time on the 10% that you *can* control, and you'll do well 90% of the time. Use negative moods as alarm clocks. Then do something about them immediately. Don't let them change from states to traits.

CHAPTER 29

When Someone You Love Is in Trouble

Here's how to know when to "butt in"— and what to say when you do

Many of us have someone in our life whose actions put them or others in harm's way—someone who is mentally ill, drinks and drives, uses illicit drugs, is in an abusive relationship, or is an abuser himself. Maybe someone specific comes to mind as you read this. Although we want to do something to help alter the course of events, we're often paralyzed by our fear that we'll be rebuffed. Or maybe we're simply not sure whether or not we know the right thing to do.

To help you decide when and how to approach someone who you believe is in trouble, top psychologists and other experts offer the following suggestions. What they have to say just may help you avert a tragedy.

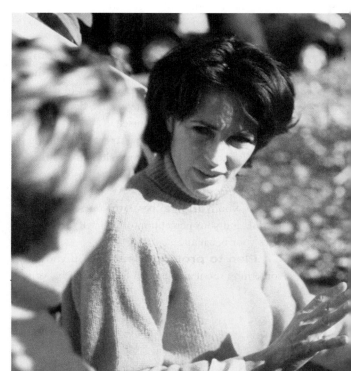

People don't have to *want* your help to benefit from it.

Overcome Your Fear

Because we're all so busy these days, we tend to see less of each other than people did when our parents were kids—which makes it harder for us to interfere. "You really have to stick your neck out to explore what's happening in your loved ones' lives," says *Prevention* advisor Edward M. Hallowell, MD, the author of *Human Moments: How to Find Meaning and Love in Your Everyday Life* (Health Communications, Inc., 2001). "It's a hassle, especially if you have an opinion that's in any way critical about what you learn. You risk enduring conflict and even rejection. And while the desire to do good is a strong impulse in people, the impulse for self-protection is just as powerful."

In fact, according to intervention facilitator Debra Jay, the number one reason that most people decline to get more involved in the troubles of friends and family is the fear that the person they aim to help will become angry and break off the relationship.

"It's a very real risk," admits Jay, a former addiction counselor based in Grosse Pointe, MI, who now helps people intervene in the troubled lives of loved ones. "But what most people don't understand is that anger isn't unavoidable. Help can be given positively, and it can be received that way too"—even, she promises, by someone who doesn't want any help.

"When someone you love has a problem and doesn't appear to want help, there is *absolutely* something you can do: You can think about what might get her to want help, then you can help her get it."

That's simply what caring friends and family members do: They stick their neck out, taking risks for others. "The thing people usually say when they're trying to convince themselves that it's okay to sidestep something that's concerning them is that it's none of their business," says Jay. "But if someone you love is having a problem, and she can't help herself, it *is* your business, because at least part of your business is loving her."

Have No Regrets

In many studies over the past decade, Thomas D. Gilovich, PhD, professor of psychology at Cornell University in Ithaca, NY, has found that Americans harbor many more regrets over inaction than action. We rue what we haven't done far more than what we've done. In fact, one of our most common regrets is not having spent enough time with loved ones.

Interestingly, a 1989 study published in *Counseling and Values*, the official journal of the Association for Spiritual, Ethical, and Religious Values in Counseling, reported "not being more assertive" and "not taking more risks" (both regrets of inaction) among the most frequently mentioned regrets.

Combine these findings, and you have a snapshot of what we have become: a vast collection of individuals who want and value connection with others, but are unable to reach out for fear that the hand we extend will get slapped. "We're so heavily influenced by the immediate sting of regrettable action that we're prone to favor inaction over action," explains Dr. Gilovich. "It's this concern with the short-term negative consequences of action that blinds us to the more enduring and painful consequences of inaction."

Make the Decision to Act or Not Act

If you have a friend or loved one you suspect may need your help but is unable or unwilling to ask for it, the experts urge you to dare to do something. Risk initial rejection in order to deepen your relationship, and come to the aid of the person you love. If you don't act, you face living with the agony of knowing you could have done something to prevent a suicide, a fatal car accident involving a drunk driver, or even a friend's broken heart. Sometimes it's easy to envision what tragedies may be looming on the horizon. But some decisions aren't so black and white.

"The hardest thing is to take that initial step, to realize that it's okay to step into another person's life if you're doing so out of love and concern," says Margo Isola. Isola, a registered nurse and manager of a surgical center in Palo Alto, CA, recently joined her three siblings in confronting their father who, after retiring at age 74, became an alcoholic. "Discussing our concerns with Dad was very, very difficult," she admits. "My father ran multimillion-dollar companies, and there we were, his kids, saying, 'You're not in control of your life.' But his behavior and health had deteriorated to the point

When "Butting In" Stopped a Killer

In February 1996, David Kaczynski, then a social worker, spent his days counseling at-risk youth, and his nights wrestling with the anguishing notion that his older brother, Ted, once a brilliant professor of mathematics, was in very serious trouble.

The previous September, the *Washington Post* had published the rancorous antitechnology "Manifesto" written by the serial mail bomber known as the Unabomber (an alias coined by the FBI, because the bomber had initially targeted universities and airlines). Three people had been killed and another 23 injured over the past 17 years. To David's ear, the wording and ideology of the "Manifesto" sounded eerily like that of the letters he often received from his brother, from whom he had been estranged for nearly 7 years.

David told Ted he wanted to see him and talk to him in person. Ted refused. With innocent lives at stake, David finally gave his brother's letters to a forensic profiler who, along with a number of other experts, concluded that there was about a 60% chance that the two authors were one and the same. "That's when I felt I had no other choice but to contact the authorities," says David. In January 1998, Theodore Kaczynski was sentenced to four consecutive life terms without parole plus 30 years.

Now, years later, David still does not feel "good" about turning his brother in. "But I know, absolutely, that it was the right thing to do," he asserts. "We live in a country that has a justifiably deep respect for the autonomy of the individual. But we as humans are profoundly connected to each other, and we should act accordingly. When you see someone who may pose a harm to himself and/or others, the question shouldn't be whether you should help him, but how."

that we felt we had to address it. And as I later found out, watching someone you love harm himself and those around him can be far more excruciating than confronting him about it."

Organize Your Thoughts

Once you've decided to act, it's important to do some serious thinking and planning before you actually approach the person who's in trouble. Here are some exercises to help you prepare for what's ahead.

Examine your motives. Before you intervene, ask yourself "Am I considering this out of love or out of envy? Out of a desire for malicious gossip? Do I want to tear him down?" If you're not sure, talk with someone else about the loved one's problem and also about your own motives. "Serious problems can be isolating," says David Kaczynski, the man who turned in Unabomber Ted Kaczynski and is now executive director of the Albany-based New Yorkers against the Death Penalty. "They can be isolating not only for the person suffering the problem but also for those trying to help. Seek out others who may also be concerned to gain some perspective, and perhaps even get some professional advice." (See "When 'Butting In' Stopped a Killer" at left for David's story.)

Shift your thinking. Instead of viewing what you're doing as butting in, which has a negative connotation, see it as creating a meaningful connection through meaningful discussion. You're going well beyond "How's the weather?" and pushing the depths of your relationship. "It's a tremendous compliment that you'd be willing to

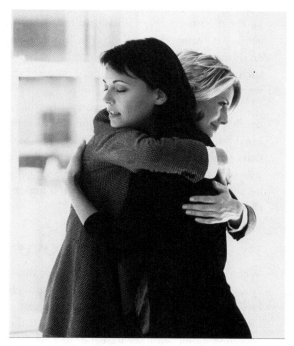

Anger is avoidable: Help can be given and received with love.

risk disfavor in order to help someone and to forge a more meaningful connection," points out Dr. Hallowell. "Think of intervening in that way, express your concerns in that way, and they may be received in that way too."

Plan the moment. Helping a friend doesn't have to feel like high stakes poker. "If you approach your loved one with the support of others and strategically plan the encounter—meaning where, when, and how it happens—you don't have to risk everything," notes Dr. Hallowell. But you do have to do it in person. "People will bring up the most incredibly difficult stuff via e-mail, because it's easier that way," he says. "But it's also disastrous: There's no tone of voice or no body language with e-mail. And you need those things when you're covering sensitive ground."

Head off defensiveness. In other words, preface any criticism with praise. Put your loved one at ease by saying "I really love you, and that's why I'm concerned." Let it be known that you may be wrong about your suspicions, but because you care so much, you thought it important to address them.

‖ Intervene with Love

When most people think intervention, they think "tough love." And when most people think tough love, they just think *tough*. Intervention facilitator Debra Jay would like to change that. She is the coauthor, along with her husband, of *Love First*

(Hazelden, 2000), the Hazelden Foundation substance-abuse treatment center's official guide for intervention. Jay has devised a kinder, gentler, and arguably more effective way of staging an intervention that hinges on love.

"I think it's a misconception that intervention has to be angry," she says. "You can use love, not confrontation, to break through the denial many people develop to coexist with their troubles. In fact, love is so powerful, much more so than anger or shame, that very little can trump it or initiate change in the same way without wounding the relationship."

Here, according to Jay, is the path that love builds.

Recruit a team. When you're dealing with someone who's very resistant to the idea that she may have a problem, you're less likely to make headway if you go one-on-one; it'll simply be your word against hers. So Jay recommends gath-

DO JUST ONE THING!

Learn to Give Up a Grudge

Forgiveness can mend more than strained relationships; it may improve your long-term health. Research has associated health risks with accumulated anger, hostility, and stress—all of which go hand-in-hand with grudge-holding. The following steps can help you get rid of any grudge you harbor. Repeat them as often as necessary until you truly are "over" it.

See it from the other side. Understand the factors that may have shaped the other person's behavior, and recognize that there are times when we hurt others too. Empathy is the gateway to forgiveness.

Acknowledge that no one can change the past. When you stop expecting that the offender can take back a hurtful act, you take responsibility for healing yourself. And don't expect an apology or changed behavior either, because forgiving doesn't equal reconciling.

Wish her well. Find a small way to genuinely wish the other person well. For example, you might say to yourself, "I hope she gains control of her temper." This helps you replace bitterness with a positive emotion.

ering a team of three to eight people, including those who mean the most to the "intervenee" (their siblings, sons, daughters, and closest friends), to approach the person.

Write down your concerns. Before the intervention, every member of the team should write their own letter to the loved one, a letter that they will read during the intervention. "The thinking is this," says Jay. "When you're doing an intervention, emotions and anxieties can run high, making it difficult to talk off the top of your head. Some people freeze, others get angry. You want to prevent both."

Edit your letter. Jay recommends following a specific, four-part structure.

1. Begin by describing what you love about the person. Mention memories, times she helped you, why you're grateful to have her in your life.

2. Note your concerns, picking two or three instances that you witnessed with your own eyes that worry you (hearsay sounds like gossip).

3. Bring love into the intervention by giving your bottom line. You might say, "If something terrible were to happen to you, and I hadn't done anything to help you, I couldn't live with myself."

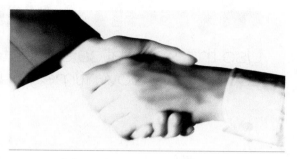

You can best convey your concern in person— not via e-mail.

4. End with a question: "Will you accept the help we're offering you here today?"

Schedule the intervention, but don't tell the person in question. "You can't notify your loved one ahead of time that you're going to intervene, because their defense mechanisms will come into play," Jay warns. "Simply invite her to dinner, or arrange to gather at her house. Then bring on the love." Regardless of what happens, at least you can say you tried.

Your Time-for-Myself Planner

Use this special calendar to make sure you get the downtime you need

Close your eyes, and imagine the one thing in the world that you'd like to do if you had more time. Now envison another. And another. Think of places you'd go, things you'd do, people you'd see, goals you'd meet, classes you'd take. Now write them on the blank lines that follow. (Don't limit yourself to 10—write down as many as you can think of.)

1. _____

2. _____

3. _____

4. _____

5. _____

6. _____

7. _____

8. _____

9. _____

10. _____